Cover Illustration: Poster for *The Raven: The Love Story of Edgar Allan Poe*, a 1909 play by George Cochrane Hazelton (1868-1921). In it, Poe is seen as an impoverished writer brooding one night over the death of his wife, when first the startling figure of a baleful raven, and then his wife's ghost, visit him. He later dies and (unlike the foreboding in Poe's poem *The Raven*), is ultimately reunited with her.

FRAGILE BRILLIANCE

THE TROUBLED LIVES OF HERMAN MELVILLE, EDGAR ALLAN POE, EMILY DICKINSON AND OTHER GREAT AUTHORS

Wallace B. Mendelson

Pythagoras Press

Printed in the United States of America.

First printing: September 2021

About the Author

Wallace Mendelson, MD is Professor of Psychiatry and Clinical Pharmacology (ret) at the University of Chicago. He is a Distinguished Fellow of the American Psychiatric Association, and a member of the American Academy of Neuropsychopharmacology. He has been director of the Section on Sleep Studies at the National Institute of Mental Health, the Sleep Disorders Center at the Cleveland Clinic Foundation, and the Sleep Research Laboratory at the University of Chicago. He is the author of twelve books and numerous professional papers. He is currently a Fellow of the Faculty of History and Philosophy of Medicine and Pharmacy at the Worshipful Society of Apothecaries, London. Among his honors have been the Academic Achievement Award from the American Sleep Disorders Association in 1999 and a special award for excellence in sleep and psychiatry from the National Sleep Foundation in 2010. More information about Dr. Mendelson's work is available in Wikipedia at https://en.wikipedia.org/wiki/Wallace_B._Mendelson and on his website at http://zhibit.org/wallacemendelson.

Contents

INTRODUCTION

The poet Emily Dickinson rarely left her home after her mid-thirties, and saw few people aside from her father. When visitors came, she was apt to disappear into her room, and those who wished to speak with her did so through a closed door. Rather than interact with neighborhood children, she would send down baskets of gingerbread from her second story window. In 1874, when she was forty-four, her father passed away. The funeral was held in the front room of their home; she did not attend, but listened from her upstairs bedroom. During these years she created some of the most beautiful lyric poetry ever written in America.

In the mid-1860s, around the time of Dickinson's growing seclusion, the painter/poet Dante Gabriel Rossetti was living alone in Cheyne Walk, London, where he surrounded himself with peacocks, wombats, kangaroos and other exotic pets. He held seances in which he tried to communicate with his dead wife, and progressively began to venture out only at night. Troubled by the effects of chloral hydrate and alcohol abuse, as well as by visual difficulties for which doctors could not find a physical cause, he remembered his past successes writing poetry. He began to think more and more about his unpublished poems which in a gesture of love he had buried with his wife. One October night in 1869 the coffin was dug up, the manuscript extracted, and the next year *Poems by Dante Gabriel Rossetti* appeared in print.

When the fifty-year-old Charles Darwin's monumental book *On the Origin of Species* was published in 1859, he was away attending to his health at a remote spa in Yorkshire. He had been living for almost two decades in a former parsonage in a small village in Kent. He led an isolated life, avoiding meetings whenever he possibly could, and suffered from gastrointestinal distress, 'lumbago' and 'rheumatism'. He had crying spells, and at other times seemed unable to speak or had mysterious paralyses. He was seen by some of the most prominent doctors of his age, who could never find a specific cause for his various symptoms, until many years later they agreed that he was suffering from angina not long before his death in his early seventies.

These remarkable individuals—as well as their contemporaries Herman Melville, Edgar Allan Poe and Nikolai Gogol—had something in common: they produced a body of extraordinarily creative work while living remarkably troubled lives. This book explores how this came about.

The notion that intellectual brilliance is somehow associated with behavior outside the conventions of society—or to frank mental illness—goes back to the very beginnings of Western culture. In the *Phaedrus,* composed by Plato in the fourth century BC, Socrates suggests that not all forms of irrational behavior are detrimental, and that indeed some types of 'divine madness' come from the gods, including the gifts of poetry from the Muses, and love from Aphrodite (Cooper, 1997). Aristotle believed that 'Poetry demands a person with a special gift for it, or one with a touch of madness...' (Barnes, 1984). This notion has continued over the centuries, and expanded to include corollaries such as a link between great writers and alcoholism. In more modern times it has persisted, with, for example, the novelist E.F. Doctorow's assertion that 'Writing is a socially acceptable form of schizophrenia' (Plimpton, 1986).

This type of thinking is so deeply ingrained that the few scholars who have argued against it have not fared well. In the 1920s, the prominent Stanford psychologist Lewis Terman argued that creative people generally had less evidence of mental disturbances or adjustment difficulties than others (Terman, 1925), only to see his work overshadowed by the rapid growth of Freudian analysis, which suggested that creativity is a method of preventing neurosis, in which artists try to deal with troubling sexual thoughts in a socially acceptable manner. When the journalist Alistair Cooke asserted that writers were troubled by alcoholism no more than plumbers, the artist and writer Barnaby Conrad responded that if this were so, 'the drains of America would be constantly clogged' (Goodwin, 1988).

In the last few decades, studies of creativity have grown into an academic discipline, embodied in periodicals such as *The Journal of Creativity* and *The Journal of Creative Behavior.* Influential books such as Kay Redfield Jamison's *Touched with Fire* (1996) have argued that manic-depressive illness (now bipolar disorder) contributed to the work of many artists. Johan Wolfgang von Goethe, for instance, has been thought to have had bipolar illness which manifested itself about every seven years, affecting his productivity for about two years each time (Steinberg and Schonknecht, 2020).

The purpose here is neither to support nor refute the admittedly fascinating endeavor of assigning specific psychiatric diagnoses to historical figures. It does grow out of my fascination with the troubled lives and peculiar behavior of a number of remarkable writers and artists, who somehow managed to produce works that have enriched all our lives. The goal here is to tell their story, and to try and give a sense of what their experiences were like.

The group selected for this book came together naturally, with the realization that a number of writers and others to whom I had always been drawn were contemporaries. Herman Melville, Edgar Allan Poe, Emily Dickinson, Dante Gabriel Rossetti, Nikolai Gogol and Charles Darwin were all born within a roughly 20 year period in the early 1800s. I've also touched on Abraham Lincoln—so depressed in his younger years that his friends sequestered his knives and sharp objects—to suggest that the troubled lives of brilliant individuals are seen far beyond the bounds of writing and art. By choosing people who lived around the same time, it is also possible to see how they influenced each other (Rossetti as a young man was drawn to Poe's writings, which may have also influenced Melville; Emily Dickinson was affected by Darwinian thought). One can also look at how they responded to the same contemporary world events (Melville attempted to save a foundering career with poetry about the Civil War, while Dickinson used the war as a vehicle for her feelings about loss).

These stories comprise what is sometimes called 'collective biography' (Mendelson, 2020), which makes it possible to see parallel experiences in the lives of the subjects. Edgar Allan Poe and Emily Dickinson, for instance, both dealt with the death of a loved one in their mid-teens, initiating themes of loss which appeared in their writings for years to come. The broader purpose is to give a sense of how such difficult lives were associated with remarkable artistic expression and production. For those who would like to pursue this further in a more academic manner, the Addendum summarizes some of the major research about the relationship of mental illness and personality traits with creative artistic expression. We will also note what is often missing when looking at writers and artists through the lens of psychiatric diagnoses. The first of these is an understanding of the influence of the social milieu, moral codes and major events of their times. The second is more elusive, but its existence comes out in the numbers—mental illness is very frequent, while great artists are exceedingly rare. It seems more likely that the various disorders and personality traits we will look at might either inhibit or predispose to brilliant creativity, depending on other qualities, and we will consider what some of them may be. In the stories presented here, one can glimpse the way they sometimes all come together, with spectacular results.

A few words about the scope of this book: As examples of creative people I have dealt primarily with writers and poets, touching on visual artists, but with little mention of the performing arts. One reason, of course, is that the technology in the early nineteenth century was such that although we have no shortage of books and paintings to look at now, we do not have recordings of performers at work. Another aspect is an intuitive sense that performing art, which often involves interpretation of the work of composers or playwrights, as well as the immediacy of interacting with an audience, may involve an equally great but somewhat different process of creativity from that of the group considered here. It could be argued that it is stretching even to consider writers of fiction and poetry together, as some researchers have suggested that poets may be more influenced by mental disturbance (Kaufman, 2011) and may have shorter lifespans, due among other things, to suicide (Kaufman, 2003). It seemed necessary to include both, however, as Melville, Poe, and Gogol wrote in both mediums.

I have touched on the visual arts as Rossetti was both a painter and poet, and his concerns and the effects of events in his life are seen on both paper and canvas. Although Darwin's fame rests with his work as a biologist and his formulation of evolutionary theory, his thinking was influenced by poetry and very much tied up with art. Indeed, the development of his ideas was likely affected by the poetry of his grandfather, Erasmus Darwin, who described 'transmutation', anticipating a theory of evolution and the descent of man. During the voyage of the *Beagle*, Darwin produced watercolors of mountains, sketches of his specimens, and later cryptic diagrams of evolutionary flow. He worked closely with artists to illustrate his books, and indeed his influence on art was commemorated in 'Drawing from Darwin', a show at the Yale Center for British Art in 2009 (Zimmer, 2009). In his later years, he was one of the first to use photographic illustrations in his books. Indeed, a willingness to cross boundaries which seem more fixed to most of us is one of the hallmarks of creativity, which is the subject of this book.

REFERENCES for INTRODUCTION

Barnes, J. (ed.): *The complete works of Aristotle: the revised Oxford Translation, Vol. 2.* (Bollingen Series LXXI-2). Princeton University Press, 1984.

Cooper, J.M. and Hutchinson, D.S. (eds.): The Phaedrus, in *Plato: Complete Works*, 1997.

Goodwin, D.W.: *Alcohol and the writer.* Andrews and McMeel, Kansas City and New York, 1988, p. 6.

Jamison, K.R.: *Touched with fire: manic-depressive illness and the artistic temperament.* Free Press, 1996.

Kaufman, J.C.: The Sylvia Plath effect: mental illness in eminent creative writers. J. Creative Behavior 35: 37-50, 2011.
https://doi.org/10.1002/j.2162-6057.2001.tb01220.x

Kaufman, J.C.: The cost of the muse: poets die young. Death Studies 27: 813-821, 2003.
http://www.stat.yale.edu/~jtc5/238/readings/cost-of-the-muse-poets-die-young.pdf

Mendelson, W.B.: *Trial by Fire: World War II and the Founders of Modern Neuroscience and Psychopharmacology.* Pythagoras Press, 2020.
https://www.amazon.com/dp/B08X1MRVXJ

Plimpton, G.: E.L. Doctorow, The art of fiction no. 94. The Paris Review 101, winter 1986.
https://www.theparisreview.org/interviews/2718/the-art-of-fiction-no-94-e-l-doctorow

Steinberg, H. and Schonknecht, P.: Goethe: a bipolar personality? Periodicity of affective states in Johann Wolfgang von Goethe as reflected by Paul Julius Mobius. J. Med. Biography 28: 174-180, 2020.
https://doi.org/10.1177/0967772017743880

Terman, L.M.: Genetic studies of genius: Vol. 1 Mental and physical traits of a thousand gifted children. Stanford University, Stanford, CA, 1925.

Zimmer, C.: Drawing from Darwin. Nature 458: 705, 2009.
https://www.nature.com/articles/458705a

CHAPTER ONE

HERMAN MELVILLE AND THE CATSKILL EAGLE

Herman Melville was born in New York in 1819, his mother from a prominent Albany family of Dutch descent and his father Allan, an importer of French dress goods. Both sides of the family had roots in the American Revolutionary War; his paternal grandfather had participated in the Boston Tea Party and served as a major in the Continental Army, while his maternal grandfather was a general known for defeating the British blockade of Fort Stanwix in the Saratoga campaign of 1777. Melville was said to be proud of his 'double revolutionary descent' (Parker, 1996).

The family business of selling French handkerchiefs, kid gloves, stockings and other goods went well in Herman's early years. His father moved the family into a series of ever-grander houses, stretching his resources but promoting the image of prosperity. By 1830, however, there were setbacks. In an effort to maintain appearances, Allan took out unwise loans, and became deeper in debt. Finally, with the rent three months overdue, he hastily moved the family to Albany. There he worked as a clerk at a cap and fur store, though he tried to give his acquaintances the impression that he was the manager. In December 1831 he was returning from a trip to New York to deal with his debts, when his steamboat was blocked by ice and he was forced to ride for two days in an open carriage in freezing weather. Shortly thereafter he developed a fever and delirium, frightening the family with his ravings, and died in late January.

After Allan's death, the oldest son, Gansevoort, set himself up in the cap and fur business. Herman, who had left school the previous year due to the family's financial difficulties, worked first in a bank and then at the store. He continued to read avidly and by 1835 was able to attend Albany Classical School, where he was particularly attracted to Shakespeare. In 1837 a financial panic led to the bankruptcy of the family business and again his withdrawal from school. He worked first on a farm, then briefly as a schoolteacher. In 1839 he studied engineering, hoping to obtain work on the Erie Canal, without success.

Unable to find steady employment, Herman followed Gansevoort's advice to go to sea. Gansevoort got him a position as cabin boy on the merchant vessel *St. Lawrence*. Four months later he returned from a round trip to Liverpool. He took a teaching position in a school which folded and failed to pay him, and unsuccessfully looked for work on his uncle's farm in Illinois. Unable to find a steady income, he signed on to the whaling ship *Acushnet*, sailing around

Cape Horn into the Pacific. A year and a half into the voyage, the harsh conditions led him and a friend to jump ship in the Marquesas Islands. There they were captured by the Typees, a cannibal tribe whose interest in him fortunately did not extend to the culinary. After a month he managed to escape on the Australian whaler *Lucy Ann*, only to be later accused of mutiny and jailed in Tahiti. He escaped once again, tried his hand at farming, and later, working as a harpooner, made his way to Hawaii. Tiring of work there as a store clerk, he enlisted as an ordinary seaman on a U.S. Navy frigate and sailed to Boston, returning to his family in 1844.

Happily, things were going better at home. Gansevoort, who had gone to law school, was now a diplomat stationed in London. With less financial pressure, Herman now had time to write. In 1846 he published *Typee*, a romanticized version of his experiences among the cannibals, and in 1847 he came out with the sequel *Omoo*, based on his voyage on the Australian whaler, the mutiny and his subsequent jailing. Both were successes, and Melville developed a reputation as a writer of adventuresome tales. Any happiness he achieved was tempered, though, by the death at age 30 of Gansevoort, who had written him a very depressive letter from London and died displaying possibly psychotic symptoms some time thereafter. Whether his excited state close to death represents mania, as some have suggested, or delirium, possibly associated with tubercular meningitis, is not known. In addition to the emotional impact, the family was now more dependent on Melville's writings. Financial pressure became even greater when he married Elizabeth Shaw, daughter of a prominent Massachusetts judge.

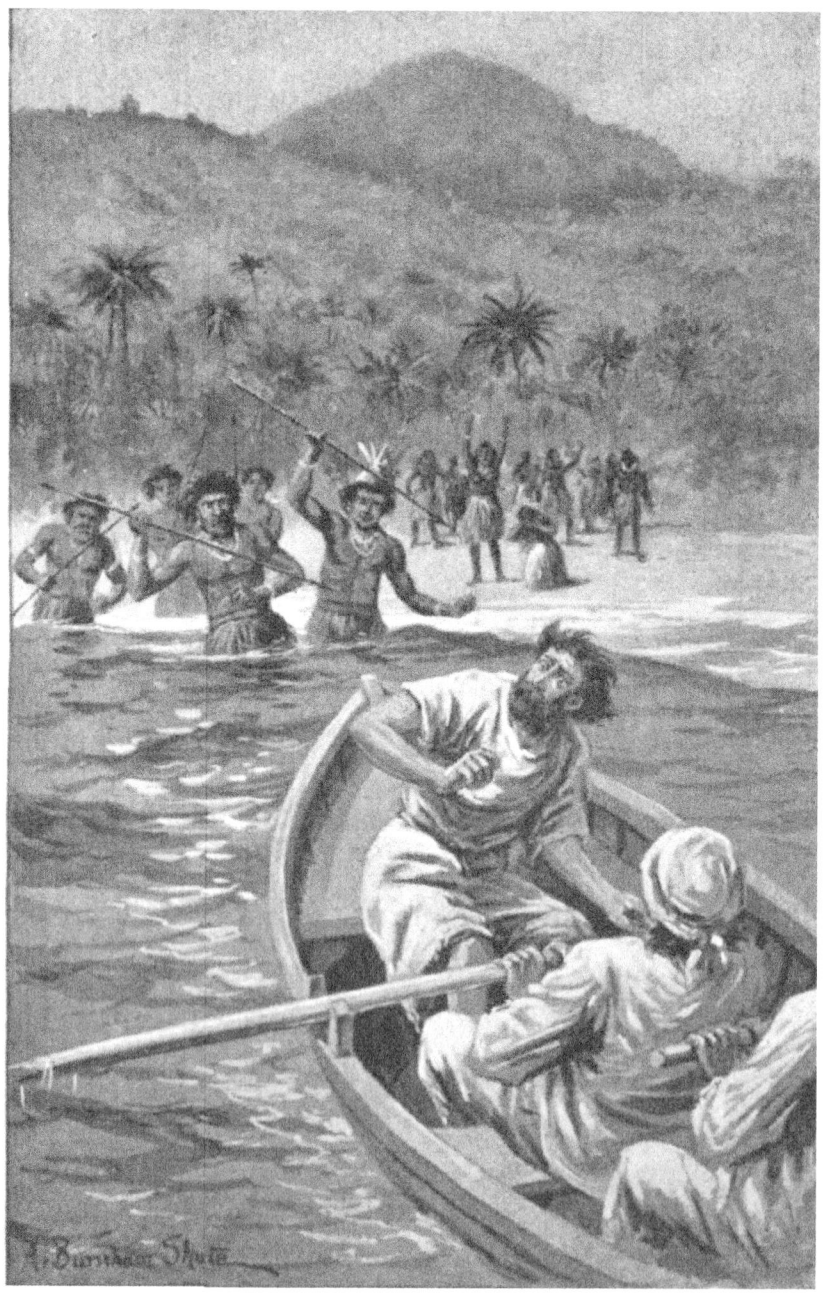

Figure 1-1: *Illustration from Melville's* Typee, *by American artist and illustrator Augustus Burnham Shute, 1892. Written when Melville was 22,* Typee *was based on his own experiences, to which he added from materials he subsequently read about the way of life of the inhabitants. It was his most well-known book when he was alive.* Moby Dick, *for which he is now best remembered, only began to be widely recognized about three decades after his death.*

Melville was also a little resentful that he was being stereotyped as a writer of adventure stories, and as if in response, came out in 1849 with *Mardi*. In its preface he commented that while *Typee* and *Omoo* were works of non-fiction about which some readers were skeptical, *Mardi* was his first work of pure fiction, which he thought readers might take to be factual. Once again centered on the exploits of South Seas voyagers, it slipped as well into the allegorical and the fantastic, describing strange lands, such as Hooloomooloo, the Isle of Cripples, and Yillah, the island of sexually innocent happiness. It left readers puzzled, and reviews were not encouraging.

In a burst of feverish energy, he tried to regain both his reputation and his finances, producing two more novels in only four months. *Redburn* recounted the experience of a young American, the son of a gentleman, among the cruder sailors in the shabbier parts of Liverpool. *White-Jacket,* based on Melville's experiences aboard the U.S. Navy frigate, described the harsh life of the crew. In a way analogous to the reaction to Nikolai Gogol's *The Government Inspector,* some readers focused on its qualities as an exposé of a corrupt governmental system, but in both cases, the authors may have had a more personal viewpoint in mind. *Redburn* and *White-*

Jacket restored the public's confidence that after *Mardi* the traditional Melville of *Typee* was back. At the same time, though, there was a darker undertone in the new books, perhaps influenced by Melville's readings of Shakespeare, notably *King Lear.*

In 1850, Melville met Nathaniel Hawthorne at a picnic, and felt he now had a kindred spirit. He had been influenced by Hawthorne's *Mosses from an Old Manse,* and in a review described it as richly 'shrouded in blackness, ten times black' (Mellow, 1980). He also praised Hawthorne in a grandiose manner, likening his work to Shakespeare's. Hawthorne's *The Scarlet Letter,* with its emphasis on the coexistence of good and evil, cemented his feelings further. He bought a farm in the Berkshires, which he named Arrowhead, allowing him to be close to Hawthorne.

At the time, Melville had already been working on *Moby Dick*, and perhaps under Hawthorne's influence, he moved beyond writing an exciting sea tale to one which took on allegorical qualities as well as exploring themes such as obsession and revenge. There is some suggestion that this re-writing of *Moby Dick* was carried out in an excited, even frenzied state, which sometimes came through in the writing, as in this passage: 'Give me a condor's quill! Give me Vesuvius' crater for an inkstand! (*Moby Dick*, Chapter 104). He worked very long hours, often forgetting to eat. He once teasingly instructed a friend to supply 'fifty fast-writing youths…because since I have been here, I have planned about that number of future works, and can't find enough time to think about them separately' (Ross,

2008, citing Leyda, 1951). The writing itself has been interpreted by some to display 'flight of ideas', rapid changes of topics often seen in episodes of mania; the plot is intermingled with digressions (Orr, 1979) which might include for instance factual material about equipment for whaling, or speculations on the meaning of colors.

Moby Dick, which came out first as *The Whale* in 1851 in London and a month later with its final title in the U.S., was not a success initially. Americans were turning westward by this time, and novels of the seafaring life had less appeal. Melville became increasingly reclusive and distressed. He began to experience a variety of difficulties including eye strain, rheumatism, back pain and sciatica. As the years went on, he was to complain frequently of visual difficulties and sensitivity to bright light. Some of his acquaintances thought these various symptoms might be caused by a kind of mental exhaustion ('neurasthenia'), which was also suggested for Emily Dickinson (Chapter five). It is also possible that they resulted from unrelated illnesses, perhaps exacerbated by long hours working by candlelight at a desk; one modern interpretation is that they all resulted from an illness known as ankylosing spondylitis (Ross, 2008).

In an attempt to recapture his standing, Melville published *Pierre* in 1852, drawing heavily from his youthful family life, and again faced critical reviews. Though only in his early thirties, he believed that he was a failure, with nowhere else to go, a feeling which was exacerbated by a fire at his publishers' offices in New York, burning much of his work. During this period he wrote several short stories, notably 'Bartleby the Scrivener', describing an office worker whose growing depression has been seen by some critics as mirroring Melville's own mood. He visited Hawthorne, then living in London, but it was apparent that their friendship had cooled. Like Nikolai Gogol nine years earlier (Chapter two), he went to Jerusalem in 1857 in the hopes of finding inspiration, which may have been the beginnings of religious interest culminating in his later writing of *Clarel* in 1876. It was in Jerusalem as well that he had one of his many episodes of eye difficulties, which he thought might be due to the bright sunlight.

Melville returned to America dispirited and in financial distress, and for several years became an itinerant lecturer on topics related to travel. He had a tradition of turning to the sea when he felt depressed, described fictionally in the opening of *Moby Dick,* and so he set sail on his brother Tom's clipper ship for a voyage into the Pacific, returning early from San Francisco. Finally in 1866 he got a position as a customs inspector in New York, which gave him some financial security for the next two decades, though it seemingly did little to improve the depressed mood which continued to haunt him. Earlier in his life he had described mood fluctuations which in *Moby Dick* he had likened to the flight of a Catskill eagle, sometimes soaring so high as to be 'invisible in sunny spaces' and at other times dropping down into the 'blackest gorges'. Though, as he noted, even when flying low, the eagle was in the mountains and still higher than birds from the lowlands, his remaining years were mostly spent in a life of isolation and often despair.

Melville turned to poetry, and in 1866 published at his own expense *Battle-Pieces and Aspects of the War.* Though later considered a classic of American verse, at the time it sold poorly—less than 500 copies in the first years—returning only half of the expense of publication and contributing further to his financial straits. By 1867 his moodiness and ill temper left his home life a shambles. The degree to which drinking contributed is not clear; some have considered him a heavy drinker while others have suggested that this has been exaggerated (Ross, 2008). His mood swings and mistreatment of his family led some to compare him to the despotic sea captains in his novels (Robertson-Lorant, 1996). At one point his wife talked of faking a kidnapping as a way of fleeing the situation. He got along poorly with his son Malcolm, who in 1867 shot himself, and was found by Melville after he failed to appear from his bedroom.

In the years that followed, Melville continued writing poetry and in 1876 came out with *Clarel* a remarkably lengthy religious work (longer than the *Iliad* or *Paradise Lost*), based on his previous trip to the Holy Land. It too, was not received well at the time. Leaving his customs job in 1885, he continued his reclusive life. He was devastated even more by the 1886 death in San Francisco of his younger son Stanwix, a seaman. In the late 1880s he began work on the prose novel *Billy Budd*, about a youthful and naïve sailor who is wrongly accused of mutiny and strikes his tormentor, accidentally killing him. Billy's acceptance of his sentence to be hanged, and the inner peacefulness with which he approached the gallows, has been taken by some as Melville's reconciliation, or perhaps resignation, to life with all its vagaries (Maxwell, 1998). The novel was uncompleted when he was felled by a heart attack in September, 1891. While decades before he had been considered one of the leading American writers, his death was largely unnoticed, and what little material appeared in the press did not go well. The New York Times obituary referred to '*Mobie Dick*', and a later article called him 'the late Hiram Melville' (Parker, 2002). His wife attempted to edit the manuscript for *Billy Budd*, but ultimately dropped the effort and stored it in a breadbox. There it languished until 1919 when it was found by his granddaughter, who sent it along to an English professor at Columbia; it was ultimately edited and published in 1924, to much acclaim.

*   *   *

Melville's afflictions have been interpreted many different ways, but the most common view has been that he suffered from bipolar disorder (Dolman and Turvey, 2011; Jamison, 1994). His family history has been taken to support this, noting that his father died "manic, insane, and bankrupt" in 1832 (Jamison, 1994). Certainly his energy, grandiosity, and unwise exuberance in financial matters are suggestive. The extreme agitation and seemingly manic behavior in the weeks before his death, however, may very well have resulted from delirium. A similar argument applies to his brother Gansevoort, who has been described as 'mad' in the month before his death at age 30 (Miller, 1975), but showed little evidence of manic behavior during most of his life, until his last weeks when fatal tuberculosis may have caused meningitis.

Clearer evidence for depression is evident in Melville's mother, maternal grandmother and a maternal uncle. A maternal aunt was committed to an asylum (Ross, 2008), and his cousin Henry was adjudged insane. Melville seemed to recognize the significance of this burden, as in passages in *Moby Dick* referring to 'the genealogies of these high mortal miseries' (Dolman and Turvey, 2011; Melville, 1992 edition). As we described earlier, his son Malcom committed suicide in 1867 at age 18 in the midst of father-son disagreements, in a sense bringing home a family history in the most personal of ways.

Turning to Melville's own history, it is clear that he had periods of intense activity, writing for instance the two novels *Redburn* and *White-Jacket* in only four months. *Moby Dick* was written in what has sometimes been described as almost a frenzy of activity, with extremely long hours and little pause for food or rest. In the period before revising it he described Hawthorne in the most grandiose of terms; as quoted above he referred to himself in a lofty manner ('Give me Vesuvius' crater for an inkstand!') and at other times, perhaps humorously, said he needed at least fifty assistants to keep track of all his future projects. His writing itself has sometimes been interpreted as 'a scattergun spray of images' approaching 'flight of ideas', and it has been speculated that such passages were written in a manic or hypomanic state, then edited later when euthymic or mildly depressed (Dolman and Turvey, 2011). At other times he was profoundly depressed, which as we mentioned earlier he likened to when a Catskill eagle descends into the 'blackest gorges'. In the years following *Moby Dick* his mood swings were much more in this darker direction. He sought solace in travel to Europe and the Holy Land, as well as on a sea voyage around Cape Horn on his brother's ship, without relief. For much of the remainder of his life he appeared depressed and irritable, a tyrant at home. His last years were spent as a dispirited recluse, though as we mentioned some have interpreted parts of *Billy Budd* to suggest some reconciliation with life.

These speculations suggest a very intimate relationship between Melville's illness and his work. One senses that depression led to his vivid descriptions of the darker parts of the human condition and how to understand evil, while hypomanic states fueled both his imagination and the energy for such prodigious and rapid output. Some have gone so far as to wonder whether, if modern treatments for mood disorders had been available, his greatest works would ever have been written. In the next chapter we will see how bipolar illness may have manifested itself in Melville's contemporary Nikolai Gogol.

REFERENCES for CHAPTER ONE

Dolman, C. and Turvey, S.: The impact of Melville's manic-depression on the writing of *Moby Dick*. Mental Health Review Journal 16: 107-112, 2011.
https://www.researchgate.net/publication/241674934_The_impact_of_Melville's_manic-depression_on_the_writing_of_Moby_Dick

Jamison, K.: *Touched with fire. Manic-depressive illness and the artistic temperament.* Simon&Shuster, New York, 1994.

Leyda, J.: *The Melville Log: A documentary life of Herman Melville, 1819-1891, Volume 1.* Harcourt, Brace and Co., New York, 1951, p. 401.

Maxwell, D.E.S.: Herman Melville, American Author. In *Encyclopedia Britannica*, 1998.
https://www.britannica.com/biography/Herman-Melville

Mellow, James R. *Nathaniel Hawthorne in His Times.* Boston: Houghton Mifflin Company, 1980, p 335.
https://en.wikipedia.org/wiki/Special:BookSources/0-395-27602-0

Melville, H.: *Moby Dick, or the Whale.* Penguin Classics, New York, 1992 edition.

Miller, E.: *Melville.* George Braziller, New York, 1975.

Orr, L.: Digression and nonsequential interpolation: the example of Melville. J. Narrative Technique 9: 93-108, 1979. https://www.jstor.org/stable/30225664?seq=1

Parker, H.: *Herman Melville: a Biography, Volume I, 1819-1851.* Johns Hopkins University Press, Baltimore, 1996, p. 12.

Parker, H.: *Herman Melville: a Biography, Volume II, 1851-1891.* Johns Hopkins University Press, Baltimore, 2002, p. 921.

Robertson-Lorant, L. *Melville: a Biography.* Clarkson Potter, New York, 1996, p. 504.

Ross, J.J.: The many ailments of Herman Melville (1819-1891). J. Med. Biog. 16: 21-29, 2008.

CHAPTER TWO

NIKOLAI GOGOL, UNDERNEATH THE OVERCOAT

Nikolai Gogol was born in 1809 in the Ukraine, then part of the Russian Empire. Just as Melville's family was proud of their Revolutionary War heritage, his family took pride in their Cossack warrior ancestry, and rather than their Russian surname of Ianovskii, had adopted the Cossack name Gogol. Both his father, a small landowner and amateur dramatist, and his mother have been described as hypochondriacs. His mother was known to exhibit mood swings, with periods of withdrawal alternating with times of euphoria, overactivity and reckless use of money. She was also known to have made extravagant statements about him, once claiming that he had participated in the creation of the railroad and telegraph.

Nikolai was sent to boarding school at age 12, where he was a shy, mediocre student, dubbed by his classmates the 'mysterious dwarf', and known for his witty caricatures in drama productions. After graduating in 1828 with a certificate making him eligible for government work in 'the rank of the 14th class', he went to St. Petersburg to make his fortune. With a grandiosity which was to appear periodically throughout his life, he sometimes said that his talents were such that they could only be appreciated in this center of culture and sophistication. St. Petersburg, however, appeared to be indifferent to his talents. When his literary ambitions and attempts to become an actor were unsuccessful, he self-published a poem he had brought with him, 'Hans Küchelgarten', describing the efforts of a romantic figure to flee a life which though idyllic, prevented him from pursuing his dreams. The scathing reviews which followed led him to franticly buy up all the copies, and to promise himself to abandon poetry.

After this early literary disaster, Gogol decided to make a new life for himself in America, an effort which he planned to finance using the money his mother had entrusted to him for the mortgage on her farm. He made it as far as Lübeck, where he changed his mind, and remained in Germany until his funds ran out. Returning to St. Petersburg, he took a series of low-level government jobs and taught history at a girls' school, while trying to restart his literary career. Things looked up with the 1831 publication of *Evenings on a Farm near Dikanki*, combining vivid descriptions of rural life with Ukrainian folklore. Among the stories in this collection was *A Terrible Vengeance*, written in the manner of folklore but apparently original with Gogol. It notably contained an intense impressionist view of the Dnieper River as well as a spacial transformation in which the people of Kiev could suddenly see a geographically impossible sight—both the Crimea and the Carpathian Mountains.

An excerpt from Gogol's description of the Dnieper River:

'Wondrous is the Dnieper in calm weather, when freely and smoothly he races his full waters through forests and hills. No rippling, no roaring. You look and do not know if his majestic breadth is moving or not, and you fancy he is all molded of glass, as if a blue mirror roadway, of boundless width, of endless length, hovers and meanders over the green world. It is a delight then for the hot sun to look down from on high and plunge its rays into the chill of the glassy waters and for the coastal forests to be brightly reflected in them. Green-curled! they crowd to the waters together with the wildflowers and, bending down, gaze into them and cannot have enough of it, enough of admiring their own bright image, and they smile to it and greet it, nodding their branches...'

From: Pevear and Volokhonsky, 1998, with permission.

Gogol was now recognized as a rising star in the Russian literary firmament, and became friendly with luminaries of the day. Though initially pleased, he later became consumed with depressive thoughts. As he often would throughout his life, he focused on vague medical illnesses which he sometimes described as incurable, and took to his bed. Later his mood shifted profoundly, and he wrote to his friend Alexander Pushkin that he planned to write the history of the Ukraine, which subsequently expanded to all of Russia, and then the world. In 1834 he managed to get an appointment teaching medieval history at the University of St. Petersburg, for which he was eminently unqualified, and after one successful lecture full of high-sounding generalizations, his performance deteriorated. His work was erratic, and he often did not show up for lectures. He was fired in 1835.

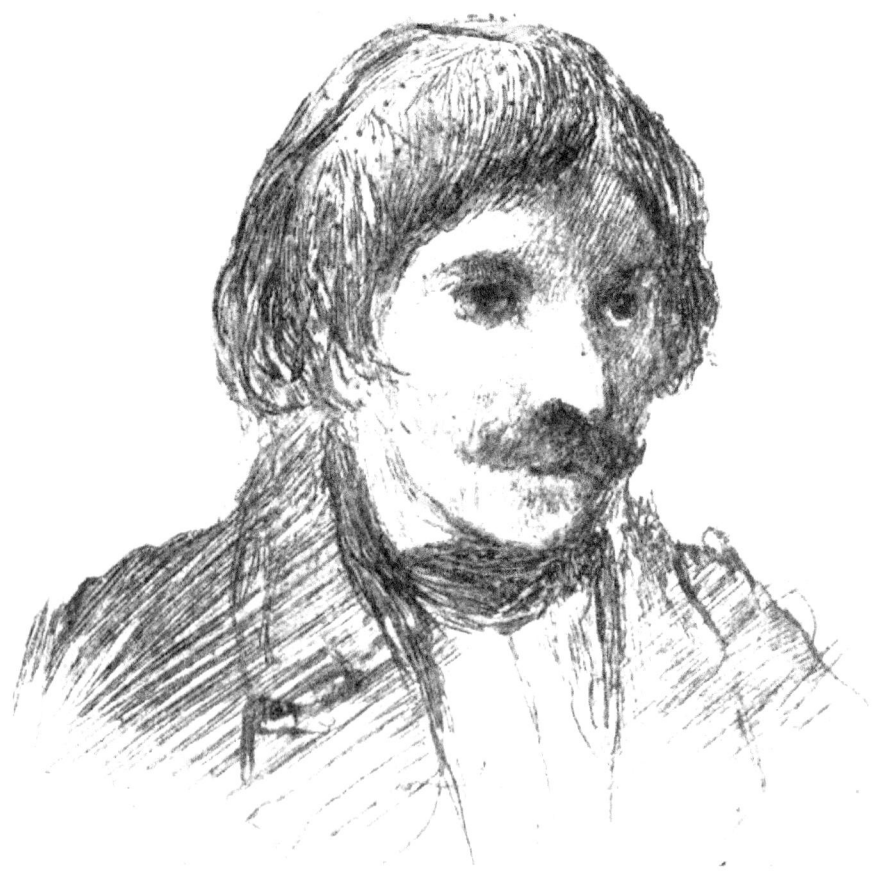

Figure 2-1: *Drawing of Nikolai Gogol by Emmanuil Dmitriev-Mamonov, 1850-1860s.*

Gogol returned his attention to his writing, which began well. Notable during these years was *Diary of a Madman* (1835), in which an office worker develops grandiose delusions, is hospitalized, and somewhat eerily in retrospect, receives treatments not unlike those Gogol was to experience years later. In *The Nose* (1836), a middling government worker awakens to find that his nose has left him, and developed a life and career of its own, with a success apparently greater than his. It marked the beginning of Gogol's insertion of the fantastic into his stories, seen in later tales such as 'The Overcoat'. It was also a precursor to later plots based on an exotic premise such as Franz Kafka's 1915 work *The Metamorphosis*, in which a man awakens one day transformed into a gigantic insect.

In Gogol's 1836 play *The Government Inspector* (1836), local small-town officials mistake a shady visitor, fond of gambling and good food but careless about paying his bills, for a government officer sent to scrutinize their work. They treat him royally in order to divert him from seeing the sorry state of their town. It is only after he has departed, and the real inspector arrives, that they realize their error. Though the production had been endorsed by the Tsar, the negative reaction of conservative critics and government officials led Gogol to flee Russia for Rome, where he largely remained for the next six years. His time there was characterized by periods of productivity in which he described himself in grandiose terms, indeed claiming powers of prophecy, and others in which he became profoundly depressed (Witzum et al., 2000). He apparently also experienced hallucinations of the seemingly supernatural (Setchkarev, 1965), which may have marked the beginning of his growing absorption in religion.

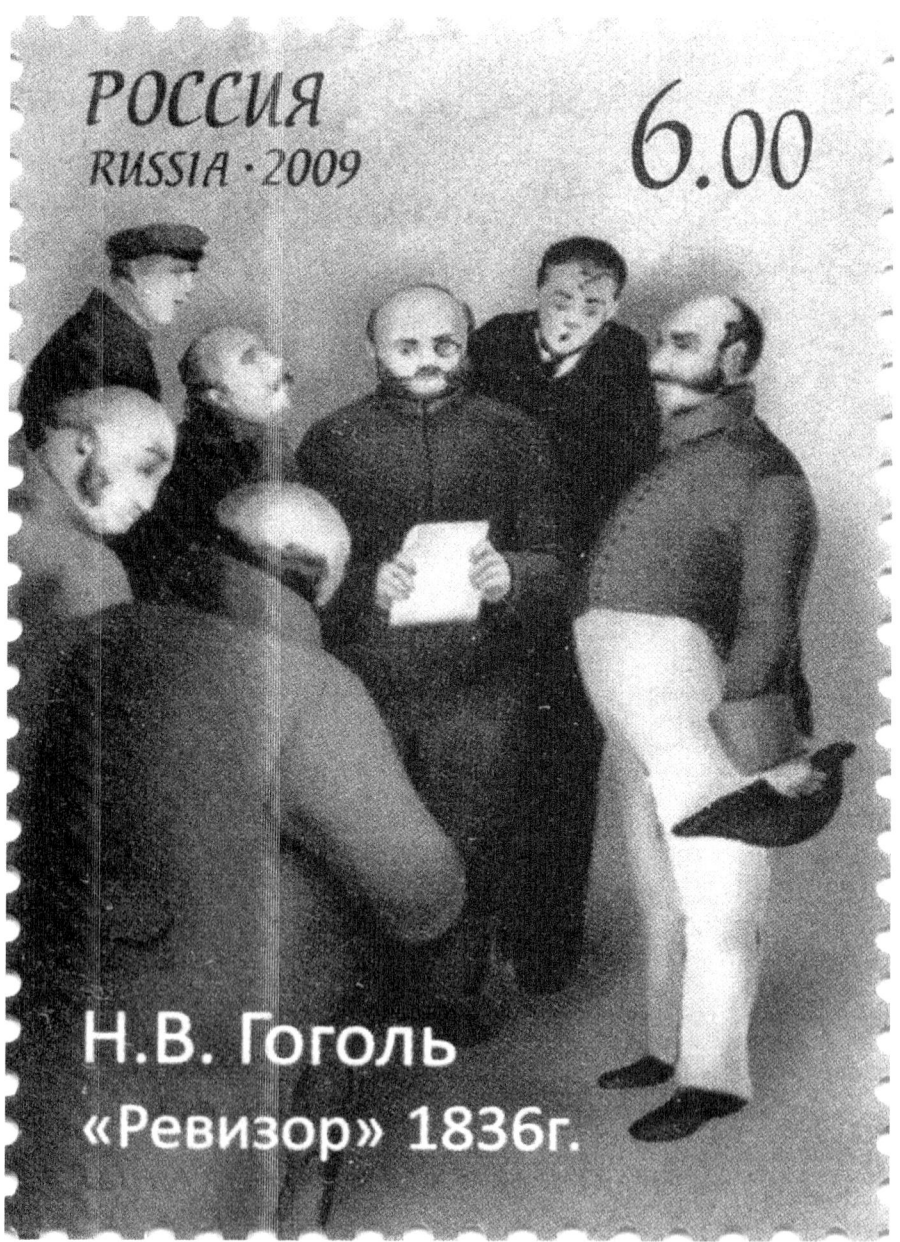

Figure 2-2: *Russian stamp picturing a scene from Gogol's play* The Government Inspector, *issued in 2009 on the 200th anniversary of his birth. Over the years it has been made into opera, dance, and films, including a 1949 version starring Danny Kaye. It was once described as one of the 15 'best plays of all time'* (The Daily Telegraph, *2014*).

During part of his time in Rome, Gogol wrote his famous short story 'The Overcoat', as well as *Dead Souls*, the novel for which he is best remembered. In 'The Overcoat', Akaky, an obscure government clerk, saves his meager earnings to buy a beautiful coat, only to have it stolen by thugs. The police are not helpful, so in his desperation he appeals to a general, only to be scorned for having brought such a trivial matter to his attention. Akaky becomes ill and dies, coming back as a ghost to haunt the city, while relieving people of their overcoats. Ultimately, he confronts the general, takes his coat, and is seen no more.

Dead Souls is the tale of Chichikov, a former government official previously fired and almost jailed for dubious transactions, with a continued interest in get-rich-quick schemes. In the novel's first section, he implements his current plan by visiting estates in the countryside and offering to buy the records of 'souls', that is, serfs, on whom the landowners must pay taxes. The catch is that he wants to purchase those who have died but are still officially listed until the next census takes place. He then plans to make money by using them as collateral for loans. The landowners, a greedy lot who are happy to rid themselves of a tax burden, wine and dine Chichikov, until word gets around that his purchases are only for dead serfs. Absurd rumors begin to appear, suggesting that he is Napoleon in disguise, or that his real goal is to run off with the governor's daughter. Chichikov flees, only to reappear with the same scheme in the second part of the novel.

When *Dead Souls* came out in 1842, it was tremendously popular. It epitomized the movement away from romanticism, which dwelled on poetic renderings of folklore and heroic figures, to realism, which told in prose the stories of contemporary, often very un-heroic characters. In this sense it paved the way for later writers such as Tolstoy and Dostoyevsky. At the same time, though, it was a work of caricature and satire of bureaucracy, with a deeper sense of the emptiness of the people he portrayed. Gogol became one of the most well-respected writers in Russia, a position vacant since the 1837 dueling death of Alexander Pushkin. Chichikov's adventures were seen by many to be a condemnation of the virtual slavery of Russian serfs, which was not abolished until almost twenty years later. Similarly, *The Government Inspector* was taken to be a condemnation of the widespread corruption in the Russian government.

By some accounts, Gogol was not fully comfortable with these social interpretations of his work (Nabokov, 1961; Merriman, 2005). He began instead to believe that God had charged him with the moral redemption of Russia, and that *Dead Souls* was meant to be only the first volume of a trilogy based on Dante's *Divine Comedy*. In his thinking, the as-yet unwritten second volume had commanded the creation of the first, which would be meaningless or even the Devil's work taken by itself (Nabokov, 1961).

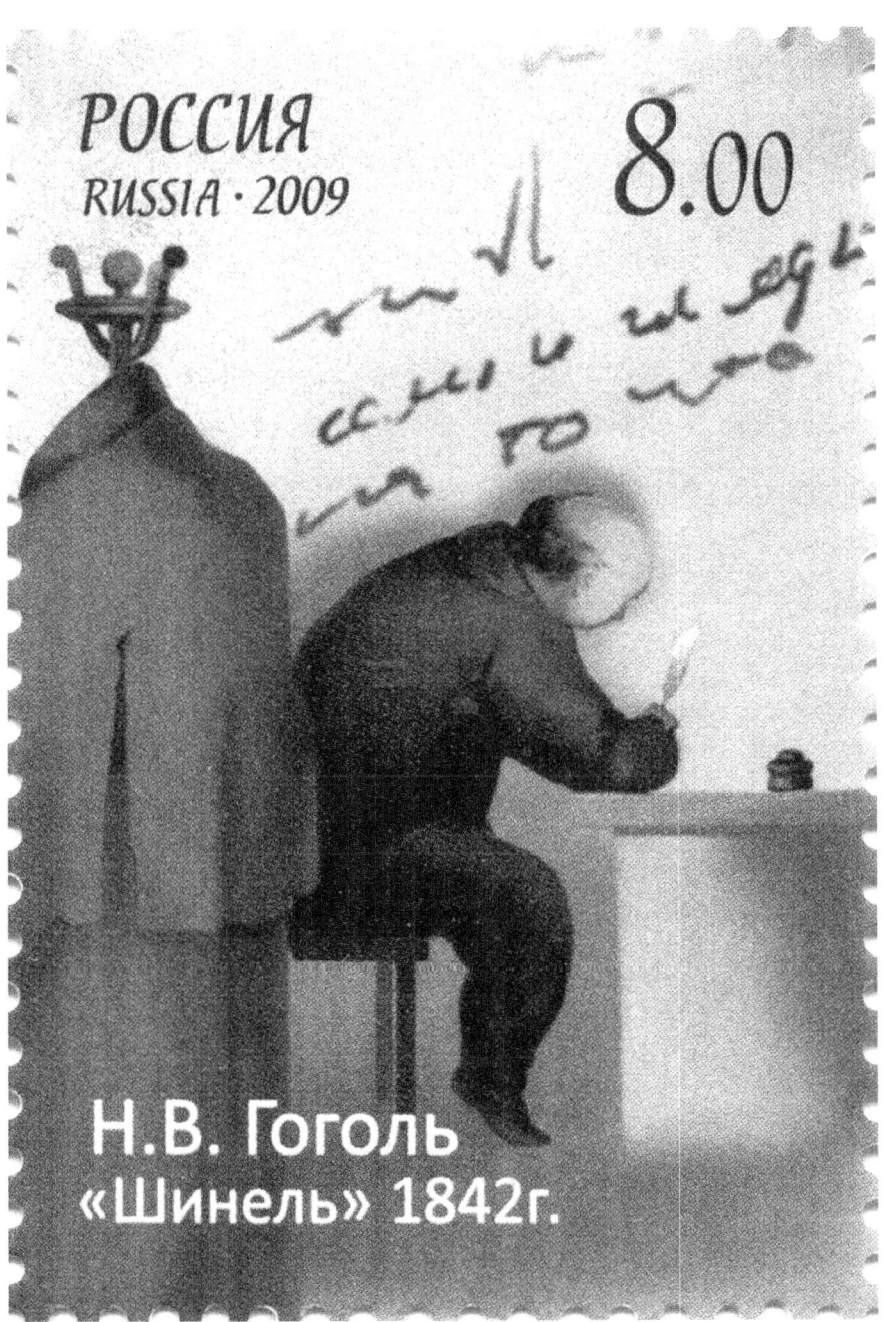

Figure 2-3: *Russian stamp showing a scene from Gogol's short story 'The Overcoat', issued in 2009. Here we see Akaky Akakievitch Bashmachkin, a middle-aged government clerk in St. Petersburg whose work is to copy letters. He is teased by his colleagues for the shabbiness of his clothes and dreams of owning a fine overcoat, with disastrous results.*

As he set about writing the sequel to *Dead Souls*, Gogol began to feel that his creative genius had left him, and the wooden portrayal of characters in the few remaining parts of the manuscript has led modern critics to share this view. At one point he burned the early drafts of the second volume. HIs interpretation was that God was sending him a new message—that instead of writing novels, he should in effect preach about sin and salvation. The result was the publication in 1847 of *Selected Passages from Correspondence with My Friends,* in which he expressed support for the Church and the Czarist regime, as well as the institution of slavery, which he asserted was supported by the Bible (Merriman, 2005). Not surprisingly, his many erstwhile supporters, who believed that he had been writing novels challenging the social system, were furious, and attacked him vehemently.

There have been many different interpretations of *Selected Passages,* and the matter is far from settled, but it seems most parsimonious to this author that Gogol was being consistent with his earlier beliefs. The conservative views espoused here had always been his, and he had written *Dead Souls* not as a denunciation of a social system built on virtual slavery, but rather as a vehicle for his specialty—the description of quirky or outrageous characters. It was also an expression of his focus on sin and the loss of one's soul in the conventional meaning of the word. Phrased somewhat differently, he may have been less concerned with the social injustice of the current system, and more focused on what he believed it did to individual's souls. He may not have anticipated that *Dead Souls* would be appropriated by those who wished to see it as a Russian prequel to *Uncle Tom's Cabin.*

Regardless of modern arguments about what may have happened, Gogol's interpretation was clear—he believed that his sins had led God to abandon him. He had feelings of hopelessness and worthlessness, and withdrew into periods of torpor so great that he worried that he would mistakenly be thought to be dead, and then be buried alive. It was rumored that he even had even wanted a coffin equipped with a rope leading to a bell above ground, which could summon help (Bernhard, 2015). He began to pray and fast more earnestly, and in 1848 set off for a visit to the Holy Land. In a letter to the poet Vasily Zhukovsky, he described his visit as having been seen 'through the mist of a dream' (Shenrok, 1892). In Nazareth he was stranded in a rainstorm, which he sat out on a bench shared with a chicken, and the experience seemed to symbolize for him the spiritual futility of the trip.

Gogol became progressively depressed, and after a period of wandering, he returned to Moscow. He continued to have mood swings, and on one occasion very inappropriately proposed marriage to a highborn countess. In desperation he sought help from

Father Matvey Konstantinovsky, a priest often described as fanatical, who subjected his hapless supplicant to 'spiritual sadism' (Lavrin, 2021). At one point Gogol began to hear voices telling him that this was the end. He fasted even more, and on February 24, 1852, he burned most of the manuscript of the later version of the second volume of *Dead Souls*, which he was convinced was the Devil's work. Exhausted and malnourished, he decided to stop eating completely and stayed in bed. A Dr. Auvers (or Hovert) undertook to treat his perilous condition. In addition to purging and bloodletting, he was put in very hot baths, followed by cold water poured over his head. He was placed in bed with leeches attached to his nose, while a muscular assistant prevented him from tearing them off. Perhaps unknowingly the doctors were feeding the leeches with an organ which had special meaning to the hapless patient, who early in his career had written *The Nose*, and sported a famously prodigious one himself (Nabokov, 1961). His worry was likely all the greater due to his longstanding fear of being buried alive. A death in panic and terror brought to an end the life of a writer whose works forged, for the first time, a truly Russian literature.

Three days after his death, Gogol was interred at the Danilov Monastery in Moscow. Seventy-nine years later, the Soviets tore down the monastery, and in the process exhumed the body in order to move it to the Novodevichy Cemetery. Stories abound that he was found lying face down, leading to rumors that he had indeed been buried alive (Cavendish, 2009). His death, like his life, continues to hold mysteries which we may never solve.

* * *

Gogol's mental state has been interpreted many different ways, including psychoanalytic studies stressing the Oedipal complex, and emphasis has been placed over the years on various aspects including possible paranoid qualities or frankly psychotic features. In his biography, Nabokov (1961), on the other hand, suggested that much of his troubled behavior could be explained by artistic *angst*. In his view, burning the manuscripts of the second volume of *Dead Souls* resulted from the tension between his artistic sensitivities and the desire to please the Church, with the realization that it was not possible to do both. Witztum, Lerner and Kalian (2000), argued that in contrast, burning the manuscripts was the result of a deep clinical depression accompanied by feelings of worthlessness and self-destructive impulses.

The notion that Gogol suffered from bipolar illness was first suggested by Bazhenov (1902), and examined in more modern terms by Witztum, Lerner and Kalian (2000), who suggested that he suffered from bipolar II disorder (see Addendum). They provided a graphic plot seeming to indicate that the number of pages Gogol wrote at various times corresponded to periods of manic behavior. An argument for some form of bipolar disorder would also come from the family history: as we described earlier, his mother was prone to mood swings from depression to periods of euphoria in which she would exhibit a great deal of energy, grandiosity and carelessness with spending money. They also suggested that Gogol might have had narcissistic personality disorder, usually thought to include an exaggerated sense of self-importance, a great need for admiration, and strong emotional reaction to criticism.

Kay Redfield Jamison (1989 and 1995) elaborated on the notion going back to the nineteenth century that some mental disorders can help release creative impulses which otherwise might have been held back. Based on her study of the lives of various luminaries, she suggested that the times in which they were most creative had many of the qualities of mania. Others have emphasized self-reports of symptoms suggesting hypomania when they were most creative, as well as cognitive qualities which are similar in the two states, such as overinclusive thinking and richness of associations (Janka, 2004). The list of writers and artists who may have had some form of bipolar disorder is long, including not only Melville and Gogol but also Virginia Woolf, Lord Byron, Johan Wolfgang von Goethe, Vincent van Gogh, Francisco Goya, George Frideric Handel, Gustav Mahler, Robert Schumann and many others (Janka, 2004). We will explore studies of the possible relationship of bipolar disorder and creativity in the first section of the Addendum.

Certainly, one caveat which must be considered is that in full-blown manic episodes, the degree of disorganization is often so great that it might preclude the control and order, which along with inspiration, are important to the creation of a novel. This is presumably the reason that some authors suggest for Gogol a diagnosis of bipolar type II disorder. This remains a matter of speculation. His personal history has been interpreted in new ways by each generation depending on the current experiences and thinking of their time, a quality his life story shares with great works of literature.

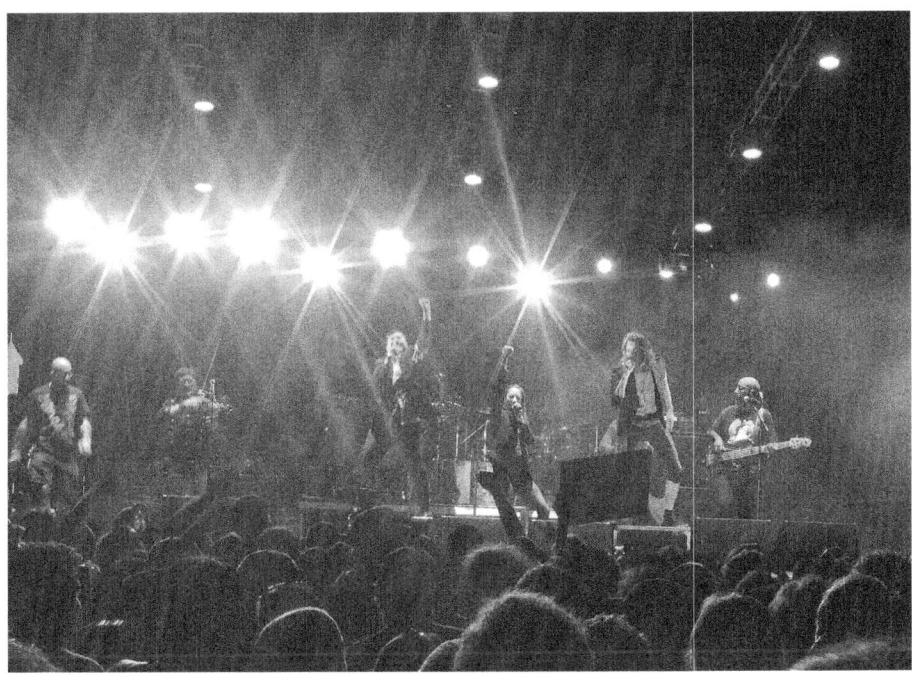

Figure 2-4: *Gogol Bordello, a punk rock band made up of an international group of musicians, performing in Baltimore in 2014. They named themselves after Nikolai Gogol because he helped introduce Ukrainian literature into mainstream Russian culture, just as the band hoped to increase awareness of Eastern European music in the West.*

REFERENCES for CHAPTER TWO

Bazhenov, N.N.: *Gogol's life and death* (in Russian). Moscow: Tovarischestvo Tipographia Mamontova, in 1902.

Bernhard, J.: Satirist Nikolai Gogol, 42, died from extreme pious pre-Lenten fasting. Dead Authors Society. April 10, 2015. http://deadauthorssociety.blogspot.com/2015/04/satirist-nikolai-gogol-42-died-from.html

Cavendish, R.: The birth of Nikolai Gogol. History Today, Volume 59, issue 3, 2009. http://www.historytoday.com/archive/months-past/birth-nikolai-gogol

Jamison, K.R.: Mood disorders and patterns of creativity in British writers and artists. Psychiatry 52: 125, 1989.

Jamison, K.R.: Manic depressive illness and creativity. Scientific American, February 1995: 46-51.

Janek, Z.: [Artistic creativity and bipolar mood disorder]. Orv. Hetil. 145:1709-1718, 2005.

https://pubmed.ncbi.nlm.nih.gov/15462476/

Lavrin, J.: Nikolay Gogol. Encyclopedia Britannica, updated February 28, 2021.
https://www.britannica.com/biography/Nikolay-Gogol

Merriman, C.D.: Nikolai Vasilievich Gogol. The Literature Network, 2005.
http://www.online-literature.com/gogol/ Accessed March 15, 2021.

Nabokov, V.: *Nikolai Gogol.* New Directions, 1961.
https://www.amazon.com/Nikolai-Gogol-Vladimir-Nabokov/dp/0811201201/ref=sr_1_10?dchild=1&keywords=Nikolai+Gogol&qid=1615744338&s=books&sr=1-10

Pevear, R. and Volokhonsky, L.: Excerpt(s) from THE COLLECTED TALES OF NIKOLAI GOGOL by Nikolai Gogol, translated by Richard Pevear and Larissa Volokhonsky, copyright © 1998 by Richard Pevear and Larissa Volokhonsky. Used by permission of Pantheon Books, an imprint of the Knopf Doubleday Publishing Group, a division of Penguin Random House LLC. All rights reserved.

Setchkarev, V.: *Gogol: His Life and Works.* New York University Press, New York, 1965.

Shenrok, V.I.: *The Facts for Gogol's Biography* (in Russian). Tipographia G. Lissner and A. Geshel, 1892-7, Moscow.

The Daily Telegraph: Best plays of all time, April 28, 2014. https://www.telegraph.co.uk/culture/books/10631419/Best-plays-of-all-time.html

Witztum, E., Lerner, V., and Kalian, M.: Creativity and insanity: the enigmatic medical biography of Nikolai Gogol. J. Medical Biography 8: 110-116, 2000.

CHAPTER THREE

EDGAR ALLAN POE, ABSINTHE AND ANNABEL LEE

Born in Boston in 1809, Edgar Poe was the son of actors David Poe and Elizabeth Arnold Hopkins Poe. His father, the son of an Irish immigrant who had been an officer in the Revolutionary War, was an actor of limited talent who was very fond of the bottle, and deserted his family when Edgar was one year old. His mother succumbed to tuberculosis a year later. The Poe children were dispersed, with his older brother Henry going to his grandfather, while his younger and mentally challenged sister Rosalie was taken in by another family. Edgar went to live with his mother's friend, Mrs. Frances Allan in Richmond, Virginia.

Mrs. Allan, with no children of her own, lavished attention on Edgar; her husband John, a well-to-do merchant, was a difficult man who withheld the praise Edgar sought from him. The family added 'Allan' to his name, but he was never legally adopted. When he was six they moved to England for five years, during which Edgar studied at a succession of boarding schools but felt isolated and never fit in very well. The family returned to Richmond and prospered due to an inheritance coming to John Allan, and these were better years for Edgar, who was known to be pleasant and was often asked to recite poetry. It was in these years that he became infatuated with a friend's mother, whom he idealized. She died when he was 15, and brokenhearted, he visited her grave regularly. Some have speculated that both his mother's death and this formative experience may have been the beginning of the theme of comely young women who die early, with a love that persists beyond the grave. His grief, however, did not prevent him from meeting, and later proposing to another young lady, Sarah Elmira Royster.

In 1826 Poe enrolled in the University of Virginia, then in its second year after having been founded by Thomas Jefferson. It was organized so that students chose their own course of studies and made their own arrangements for lodging. Many took advantage of a system which had no exams and depended on student reports of disciplinary issues, and Poe was among them. Though his skill at poetry and painting was recognized, he also earned the reputation of a reckless gambler and heavy drinker. It was said that he drank his whiskey copiously and straight, but without seeming to take pleasure in it. In less than a year his debts were so great that his stepfather paid them off but would not let him go back to the university.

Poe's return to Richmond was, not surprisingly, an unhappy one, made worse by the news that Ms. Royster had married someone else. He moved to Boston where he worked part-time as a newspaper writer, but financial pressures led him to join the army in May of 1827, using a false name and claiming that he was 22 instead of 18. He was stationed in Boston, where in 1827 he published his first book, the poetry collection *Tamerlane and Other Poems,* which met with little success. Later he was transferred to Charleston, where he was assigned to assembling artillery shells. Though he did well, rising to the non-commissioned rank of sergeant major, he tired of it. He appealed once again to his stepfather, who at the time was occupied with the illness of his wife. After her death in February 1829, he reluctantly paid the fees necessary for Poe to leave before his enlistment was over, in the hope that he would later attend West Point, to which he had used his influence to obtain an appointment.

After his discharge, Poe went to Baltimore, where he moved into the home of his 39-year-old aunt Maria Clemm, who would become a mother figure to him in time. Living there as well were her daughter Virginia, later to become his wife, as well as his brother Henry and his grandmother. During this period in 1829 he published another book of poetry, *Al Aaraaf, Tamerlane and Minor Poems* without notable success. In July of 1830 he entered West Point, in perhaps his last attempt to please his stepfather. In his seven months there he became known both for his fondness of brandy, and (like Gogol in his schooldays) for his satirical productions about his superiors.

At one point Poe's fellow cadets took up a collection to help pay for publication of more poems. If they were expecting additional biting caricatures, they may have been disappointed; it was a series of romantic works which included some of his earlier writing but also what were to be become some of his best poems including 'City by the sea', 'Israfel', and 'To Helen'. Once again Poe tired of his occupation, but his stepfather, to whom he was now estranged, would not pay the fees necessary for his release. In response, Poe refused to go to classes or church or to carry out other orders. As was his intent, he was court-martialed, and dismissed from the service.

In 1831 he returned to Maria Clemm's home in Baltimore. Not long afterwards his brother Henry died, apparently of tuberculosis but complicated by debilitation from alcoholism. While mourning the loss of yet one more important figure in his life, Poe began writing short stories to help pay the family's expenses and subsidize his poetry; it is likely that some of his income was consumed subsidizing his drinking as well. He achieved some success with the short story 'MS. Found in a Bottle' in 1833. It led to him landing a job at the *Southern Literary Messenger,* first as a part-time contributor, then as a regular writer and book reviewer, and later as its editor. He was then 26, and it was the first step in a literary career that would be cut short by his death at 40. He persuaded his young cousin Virginia, then 13, to marry him, and initially was diligent and avoided drinking. He became known for the vigor with which his reviews denounced the works of the literary stars of his day, and somewhere along the line he took up the bottle again. It led to his being fired, the first of many jobs which would end this way.

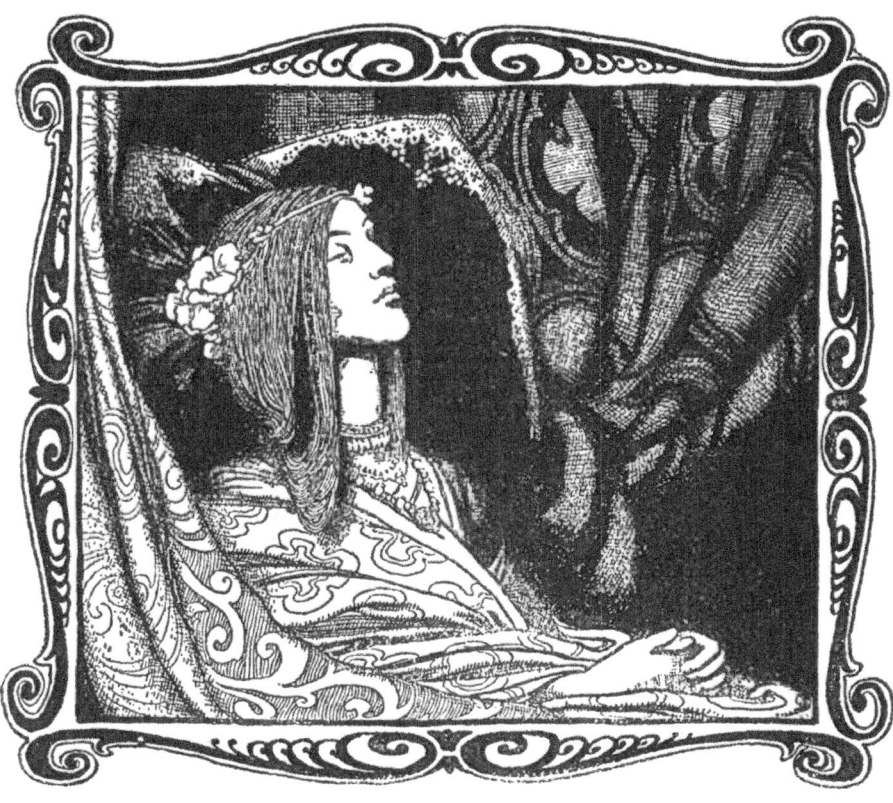

Figure 3-1: *Illustration from Poe's poem 'The Sleeper' drawn by W. Heath Robinson (1872–1944). This lyric poem, which first came out in 1831, was revised and published again in 1836 and then later in 1845, the same year as the much more famous 'The Raven'. Poe's comment on 'The Sleeper' was that 'In the higher qualities of poetry, it is better than 'The Raven'—but there is not one man in a million who could be brought to agree with me in this opinion.'* (Correspondence with George W. Eveleth on December 15, 1846). The illustration appeared in The Poems of Edgar Allan Poe (George Bell & Sons, New York, 1900).

Poe moved from city to city, working briefly at various newspapers or journals before being let go, and freelanced his stories and poems. He became notorious for appearing drunk in public, but his productivity continued. In 1835 he came out with 'The Unparalleled

Adventure of One Hans Pfaall', involving a balloonist who travels to the moon, which may have influenced Jules Verne's later *From the Earth to the Moon*. In 1838 he published the novel *The Narrative of Arthur Gordon Pym of Nantucket,* which began as a sea saga; indeed it has been thought to have influenced Melville's writing of *Moby Dick* (Quinn, 1952). Like many of his tales it evolved into the fantastic, including the 'hollow Earth theory' (contributing further to the claim that he was one of the fathers of science fiction). In 1839, while an editor at *Burton's Gentleman's Magazine* he published 'The Fall of the House of Usher', which like many of his tales dealt with being buried alive, a fate very worrisome as well to Nikolai Gogol (Chapter two).

In 1841 Poe moved on to *Graham's Lady's and Gentleman's Magazine,* where he published his story 'The Murders in the Rue Morgue', which may have been the world's first modern detective fiction. He won a $100 prize for 'The Gold Bug' in a contest sponsored by the *Dollar Newspaper* of Philadelphia. He moved, once again, to the *New York Mirror,* where he published his poem 'The Raven', securing his reputation. His career—and his drinking—continued as he moved from job to job, writing not only his stories but also gossipy pieces about the luminaries of the day which often landed him in trouble. His behavior became more erratic as time passed. On one notable day he was drunk and failed to arrive for an appointment with President Tyler, who was prepared to discuss the possibility of steady work in the government. He often took to his bed with ill-defined disorders in a manner reminiscent of his contemporary Charles Darwin (Chapter six), and sometimes feared that, like his wife, he may have contracted tuberculosis.

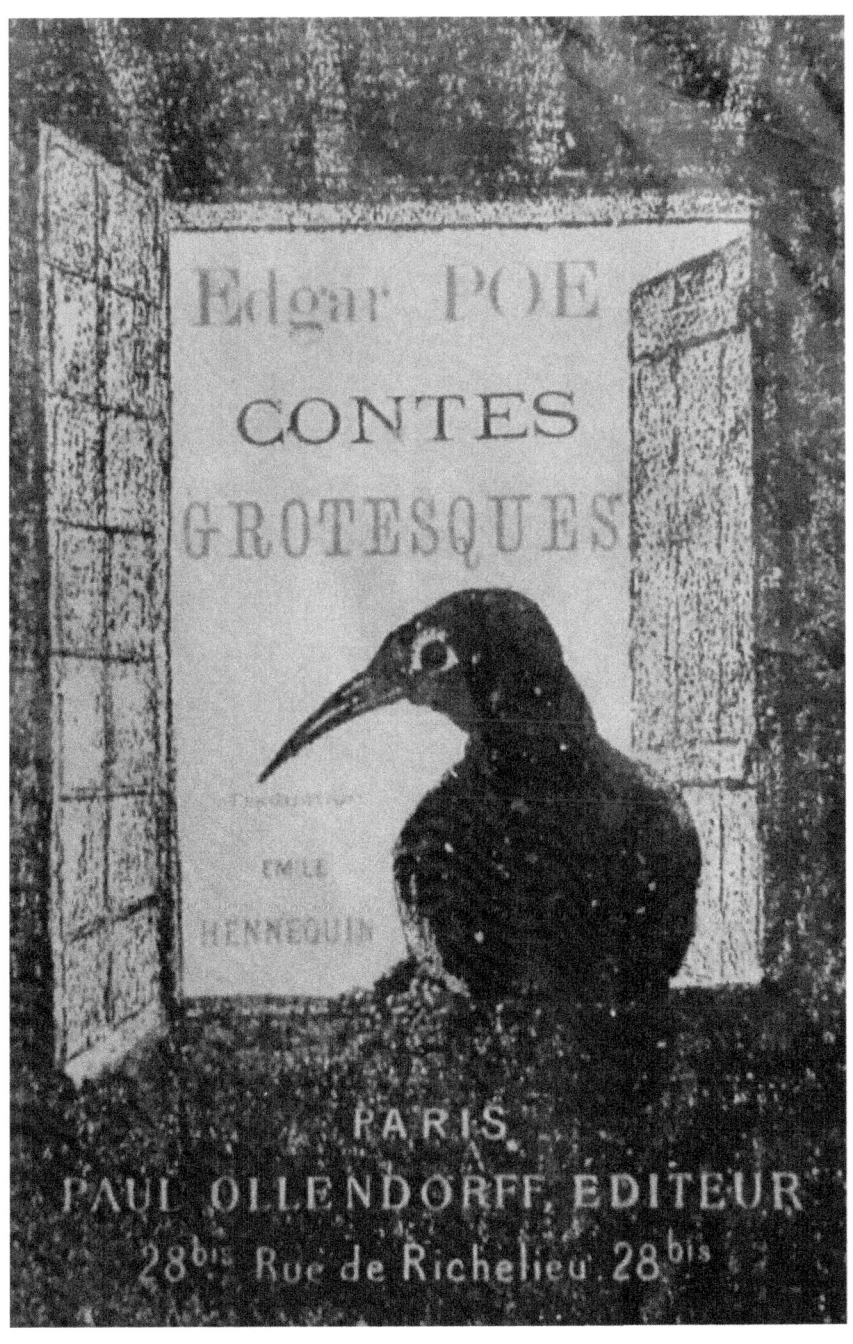

Figure 3-2: *French edition of Poe short stories, published in Paris by Paul Ollendorff, 1882. The cover painting of the raven was by Odilon Redon (1840-1916), whose later 'dreamlike' paintings were thought to have influenced the development of Dadaism and Surrealism.*

Poe's complex relationships with women continued as well. In 1845, correspondence from the poet Frances Sargent Locke Osgood surfaced; though Virginia had been aware of this chaste romance and viewed it with acceptance, the resultant publicity caused quite a scandal. After Virginia died in 1847, Poe pursued several other women with great ardor which remained chaste and usually resulted in new poems about them. At first he thought he could control his drinking, writing 'I had indeed, nearly abandoned all hope of a permanent cure when I found one in the death of my wife.' (Letter to George W. Eveleth, January 4, 1848; Delphi Classics, 2011). His abstinence was short-lived. He often disappeared for days at a time, and the extreme degree of intoxication manifested in public led to rumors of drug use as well. He began to have trouble concentrating and suffered from headaches, which he described in his poetry.

After a particularly notable drinking bout in Philadelphia in 1849, Poe returned to Richmond. There he reconnected with Elmira Royster, the sweetheart of his younger years, now widowed. He wooed her and she agreed to become engaged once again, with the stipulation that he stop drinking. Though he made some efforts, it was not to be. He left for a trip to Baltimore, where he went missing for several days before being found in a tavern, stuporous and wearing someone else's clothes. In his final days in the hospital he was delirious, agitated and hallucinating, calling out for 'Reynolds' (who has never been identified). Like Darwin, he was buried in Westminster, but in this case it was Baltimore's Westminster Presbyterian churchyard. Two days later his last poem, *Annabel Lee*, commemorating his love for his deceased wife, was published by the *New York Tribune*. Unlike the hopelessness of *The Raven*, it expressed the belief that they would be reunited in the next world.

*   *   *

Poe had been known for his heavy drinking going back to his college days. It had a driven, relentless quality, and did not necessarily seem to give him pleasure. He wrote 'I have absolutely no pleasure in the stimulants in which I sometimes so madly indulge. It has not been in the pursuit of pleasure that I have periled life and reputation and reason. It has been the desperate attempt to escape from torturing memories, from a sense of insupportable loneliness and a dread of some strange impending doom.' (Marsden, 1988). About two years before his death he elaborated further on drinking as an escape: 'As a matter of course, my enemies referred the insanity to the drink rather than the drink to the insanity.' (Letter to George W. Eveleth, January 4, 1848; Delphi Classics, 2011).

Poe's favorite substances were whiskey, brandy and absinthe. His friends were struck by the wild, delirious behavior which he manifested while drinking. He acknowledged his hallucinatory states this way: 'Fill with mingled cream and amber, I will drain that glass again. Such hilarious visions clamber Through the chamber of my brain — Quaintest thoughts — queerest fancies Come to life and fade away; What care I how time advances? I am drinking ale today.' (Delphi Classics, 2011).

The psychiatrist Donald Goodwin (1988) raised the interesting point that Poe's excited, delirious states occurred during his drinking, rather than during withdrawal hours or days later, which would have been characteristic of delirium tremens. He argued that this may have resulted from Poe's fondness for absinthe, sometimes called 'the green fairy' which, unlike more typical alcohol drinks, additionally contains herbal substances that can induce agitated delirium and hallucinations. (Indeed, its predilection for toxicity led to it later being prohibited in most countries.) He also noted that these are not typical symptoms of opium, which tends to produce 'a state of profound passivity'.

Whether Poe was also addicted to opium is an ongoing matter of debate (Goodwin, 1988). On the one hand, a cousin and his sister said that he used it frequently; on the other hand, two physicians who were well acquainted with him, as well as a number of friends, believed this was not the case. Opium certainly appears in many of his stories, though it has been argued that the effects he ascribes to it do not resemble typical opium intoxication or withdrawal symptoms. In those years laudanum (opium dissolved in alcohol) was a legal and easily available medicine for gastrointestinal disturbances (Mendelson, 2020), though of course often used recreationally. The English historian Alethea Hayter, who looked at substance abuse in a number of writers in *Opium and the Romantic Imagination*, believed that whether Poe was addicted to opium cannot be determined (Hayter, 1968).

It is uncertain whether Poe's description of drinking was a way of fleeing 'torturing memories' as he asserted, or whether this represented a kind of romantic rationalization. Whatever its source, his drinking led to erratic behavior which cost him his jobs time after time, later affected his concentration, and ultimately contributed to his death at age 40. As such, he is often seen as a romantic, tragic figure. Alethea Hayter made the intriguing comment that 'Everyone who writes about him chooses their own Poe' (Hayter, 1968; quoted in Goodwin, 1988). Some have seen him as driven by a need to please a cold father figure, or struggling to come to grips with the untimely deaths of his mother and wife, or of being caught between the simultaneous attraction to and fear of women. As we will note in Charles Darwin's history (Chapter six), one has the sense that he often appeared to be a mirror in which authors see reflections of their own interests or theories. One point on which most can agree, though, is that whether by intent or not, he left a legacy of the image of the brilliant, but troubled and alcoholic, writer.

REFERENCES for CHAPTER THREE

Delphi Classics: *The Complete Works of Edgar Allan Poe (Illustrated.* Delphi Classics, 2011.
https://www.amazon.com/Delphi-Complete-Works-Edgar-Illustrated-ebook/dp/B004YNIS3A

Goodwin, D.W.: *Alcohol and the writer.* Andrews Mcmeel, 1988.
https://www.amazon.com/Donald-W-Goodwin-1988-11-16-Hardcover/dp/B004RI7QWQ

Hayter, A.: *Opium and the Romantic Imagination.* Faber & Faber, 2015.
https://www.amazon.com/Opium-Romantic-Imagination-Alethea-Hayter-ebook/dp/B010KNF6QE

Marsden, S.: *Visions of Poe.* Knopf, 1988.

Mendelson, W.B. : *Nepenthe's children: the history of the discoveries of medicines for sleep and anesthesia.* Pythagoras Press, 2020.
https://www.amazon.com/Nepenthes-Children-discoveries-medicines- anesthesia- ebook/dp/B08H4XDZBN/ref=sr_1_1?dchil

d=1&keywords=nepenthe%27s+children&qid=1620922734&s=digit
al-text&sr=1-1

Quinn, P.F.: Poe's imaginary voyage. Hudson Review IV (Winter, 1952), p. 585.

CHAPTER FOUR

DANTE GABRIEL ROSSETTI AND THE WOMBAT'S LAIR

Dante Gabriel Rossetti was born in 1828 in London, a few years after his father fled the Kingdom of the Two Sicilies when his support of a constitutional government put him in the king's poor graces. His father, a poet and scholar who studied Dante Alighieri, taught at King's College London, and he grew up in a genteel family steeped in university life, with three siblings who later became respectively a poet, writer and critic. Torn between his interests in poetry and painting, and drawn to Italian medieval art, he went to King's College School, a private drawing academy, and then the Royal Academy. As a young man he read widely, including the Bible and Shakespeare, and was particularly attracted to the gothic tales of Edgar Allan Poe (Chapter three). He wrote poetry and translated Italian works into English. He was much influenced by the romantic poets William Blake and Lord Byron, and took to heart Blake's criticisms of English academic painting as exemplified by Sir Joshua Reynolds. The painters William Holman Hunt and John Everett Millais became his close friends, and together in 1848 they founded what became known as the Pre-Raphaelite Brotherhood.

The Pre-Raphaelites rejected what they considered to be the artificial techniques taught at the Royal Academy of Arts, in favor of the styles of the late medieval Gothic and Early Renaissance. They believed that bright colors and attention to detail as well as elaborate composition would lead to a return to 'truth to nature'. Rossetti brought to the movement an interest in poetry and social implications, as well as an idealized medieval past. Many of the paintings arising from the movement at that point had Biblical themes, and in 1850 at age 22 Rossetti exhibited *Ecce Ancilla Domini*, depicting Mary as a young woman. It, and many other early Pre-Raphaelite paintings, was met with fierce reviews. Like Nikolai Gogol (Chapter two), Rossetti was very sensitive to criticism. Gogol's response at about the same age to the poor reception of his first published poem had been to buy up all the existing copies, which he burned, and vow to write poetry no more. Rossetti's reaction was no less severe. He chose to work in watercolors, for which there was a private market not requiring exhibitions, and he changed from Biblical scenes to subjects inspired by literary figures such as Dante and Shakespeare.

Around this time the original Pre-Raphaelite group was falling apart, undone by the differing personalities and agendas of its members. By 1856 Rossetti had made the acquaintance of Edward Burne-Jones and William Morris, with whom he re-founded the movement in somewhat revised form. Instead of emphasizing 'truth to nature', they turned to a romanticized past exemplified by the legends of King Arthur. Under Morris's influence they also expanded their interests from painting and poetry into decorative arts and design.

Rossetti's personal life was changing as well. In 1851 he had acquired a new muse, Elizabeth Siddall, a poet and painter who first modeled for all the Pre-Raphaelites. She notably posed for Millais' 1852 portrayal of Shakespeare's Ophelia, who drowned in a brook, by lying in a bathtub during a chilly winter. When the painter's promised heating system did not suffice, she developed pneumonia, and under threat of lawsuit he covered her medical expenses. She had also been modeling for Rossetti, and after recovering she began studying with him as well; they became close and were married in 1860. It was a passionate relationship, and the intertwining of both art and love was such that he is thought to have produced more than a thousand paintings and sketches of her. After their marriage they turned inward, seemingly preoccupied with themselves and excluding the outside world.

There were also signs of difficulties in those years. Rossetti found himself protecting her from his family's criticism of her modest background (her father sold cutlery). She was chronically ill, and indeed had had to be carried to her own wedding just a short distance from their lodgings. She became addicted to laudanum, a tincture of opium (Mendelson, 2020a), perhaps as a result of treatment for her conditions, which have been speculated to include tuberculosis or anorexia.

In 1861 Elizabeth had a stillbirth and afterwards became severely depressed. Later in the year she became pregnant once again. One evening in February 1862 Rossetti returned from teaching to find her unconscious from an overdose of laudanum, though whether intentional or not has never been clear. Despite the efforts for four doctors, she passed away early the next morning. The grief-stricken Rossetti had her laid to rest in Highgate Cemetery, after placing in her coffin the manuscripts of all his unpublished poetry. By the following year he had used his many sketches of her in painting *Beata Beatrix* (Saint Beatrice), who represented perfect love in Dante's *The Divine Comedy*. She is portrayed with a red dove, thought to symbolize love, as well as a white poppy, referring to the opium which led to her death.

After Elizabeth's death Rossetti moved into a new home in Cheyne Walk, Chelsea, where he was to remain for most of his life. Since 1860 he had taken up oils again, and painted colorful, sensuous but highly stylized portraits of beautiful women. Gone was the medievalism, replaced by a style which echoed painters of the Italian High Renaissance. His work was initially successful, enabling him to fill his home with elaborate decorations and exotic animals such as peacocks, armadillos, wombats and kangaroos. Wombats were his favorites, and he sometimes invited friends to spend time with him at the 'wombat's lair' at the zoo in Regent's Park. Like Edgar Allan

Poe (Chapter three) he began to be seen inebriated in public, and by the mid-1860s was becoming more and more of a recluse, venturing out only at night. He became involved in spiritualism, and held seances in which he attempted to talk to Elizabeth.

Like Melville (Chapter One) Rossetti began to believe that his eyesight was deteriorating, though the cause has never been clear. As a result, he began to focus more on poetry. He remembered his earlier successes translating Italian verses, and thought of his manuscripts buried with Elizabeth. In 1869 he agreed to let Charles Augustus Howell, a questionable art dealer and probable blackmailer, open the coffin and retrieve the manuscripts. The following year they were published as *Poems by Dante Gabriel Rossetti*. Initially the book seemed a success, and Rossetti's health improved, with less difficulty with sleep and eyesight. Then things took an unexpected turn. A critic, Robert Buchanan, offended at the erotic content, strongly criticized the work as being what he called 'The Fleshly School of Poetry'. Stung, Rossetti unwisely responded in print, which led to even more publicity and distress.

Rossetti was sleeping poorly, and in 1869 had been introduced by an American journalist acquaintance to the newly available chloral hydrate (Mendelson, 2020a). He began combining it with whiskey to cover its strong taste or increase its effects. He and his colleague William Morris rented a house in Oxfordshire, and for a few years he spent time there with Morris and his wife Jane, who had been modeling for him for some time. He and Jane stayed there alone in the summers of 1871 and 1873 while Morris traveled.

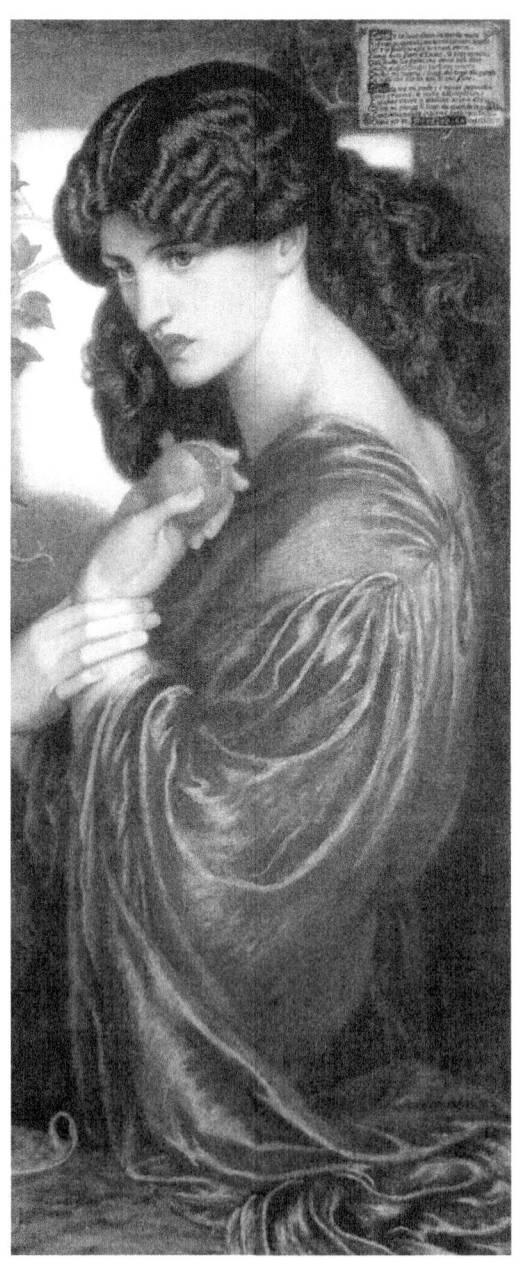

Though Rossetti continued to write and paint, his friends began to be alarmed at his lack of care for himself, occasional incoherence, and thoughts that enemies were plotting against him. In 1872 he took an overdose of laudanum; following his initial recovery, he spent time in Scotland to heal (as had Darwin before him; see Chapter six), but afterwards became even more reclusive. By 1874 his deterioration was such that Morris removed him from their decorative arts firm and the complicated relationship of the Oxfordshire years came to an end.

Figure 4-1: *Rossetti's Proserpine, 1874, for which Jane Morris was the model. In classical mythology, the goddess Proserpine (Roman) or Persephone (Greek), lived six months a year in the underworld as the wife of its king, Pluto (Hades), returning to the living world each spring. Her appearance, and then return to the underworld each fall, came to represent the yearly agricultural cycle, and in a broader sense, growth, death and rebirth.*

As time went on Rossetti's behavior became more erratic, and the women in his life, Jane Morris and his longstanding model and lover Fanny Cornforth, distanced themselves, though maintaining some contact. At times he resisted his addiction, taking long walks at night, and he underwent an unsuccessful treatment with hypnosis. He tended to sleep during the day, spending his nights imbibing whiskey and chloral hydrate. He was described as depressed, taking no pleasure in momentary bright spots such as the sale of a painting. He was now using opium as well. In 1881 he suffered a stroke limiting his ability to walk, and was thought to have been suffering from Bright's disease (chronic nephritis). On Easter Sunday in 1882 he passed away at a friend's seaside bungalow in Kent. Perhaps remembering what had taken place at Highgate Cemetery, he had asked to not be buried with his wife, and chose instead to be interred in the local graveyard.

* * *

An accident of history allows us to pinpoint the timing of chloral hydrate abuse in Rossetti's life. Though it had been synthesized in the 1830s, its development as a clinical drug began with the German pharmacologist Otto Liebreich in 1869, who demonstrated its sedative effects on medical and psychiatric patients (Mendelson, 2020a). There was a great deal of interest in its possible benefits for a variety of conditions including controlling agitated behavior in asylums and treating delirium tremens; later, the well-known Austrian psychiatrist Richard von Krafft-Ebing suggested it might be useful in psychoneurosis. Some of the enthusiasm was because it was the first sedative created by chemical synthesis, rather than by extracting from plants. As such, it was possible to have greater precision in dosing than with natural substances such as morphine, and unlike morphine, injections were not necessary. Initially, the many downsides of chloral hydrate including addiction and a medically serious withdrawal syndrome were not yet recognized. As mentioned earlier, it was in 1869, around the time of its first clinical use, that an acquaintance introduced it to Rossetti. He was to be one of many historical figures who suffered from its misuse. A few years later, Mary Todd Lincoln, Abraham Lincoln's widow, developed psychotic behavior, likely due to chloral hydrate misuse, leading to her commitment to an asylum in 1875 (Mendelson, 2020b). Nor was this confined to the 19th century; in 1953 a combination of chloral hydrate and alcohol contributed to the death of the singer Hank Williams, in the back seat of a car on the way to a concert in Ohio.

Though Rossetti and Edgar Allan Poe, whose work he much admired, suffered deterioration at relatively early ages, the arcs of their lives and the interactions of their personalities with their addictions were very different. Both were heavily influenced, though in different ways, by father figures: Poe spent much of his young life in a vain effort to please his step-father, while Rossetti inherited his father's love of Dante's poetry and medievalism which shaped his career. Poe was known for heavy, relentless drinking from his college years through most of the rest of his life; Rossetti came across chloral hydrate when an established artist at about age 41. Finally, Poe died among strangers, in unclear circumstances. In contrast, despite Rossetti's efforts, his friends and family remained faithful to him till the end. His mistress Fanny Cornforth, previously distanced due to the consequences of his drug use, returned to offer support in 1881. The bungalow in which he died in 1882 had been lent to him by an architect friend in the hope that he might convalesce there, and he was attended by his mother, brother and sister.

Rossetti had continued to paint until his last years, and published two books of poetry, an updated *Poems* as well as *Ballads and Sonnets,* in the year before his death at age 53. He had spent years evolving from one style and subject matter to another, and one wonders where he might have gone had not chloral hydrate, opium and alcohol played such a big role in his life.

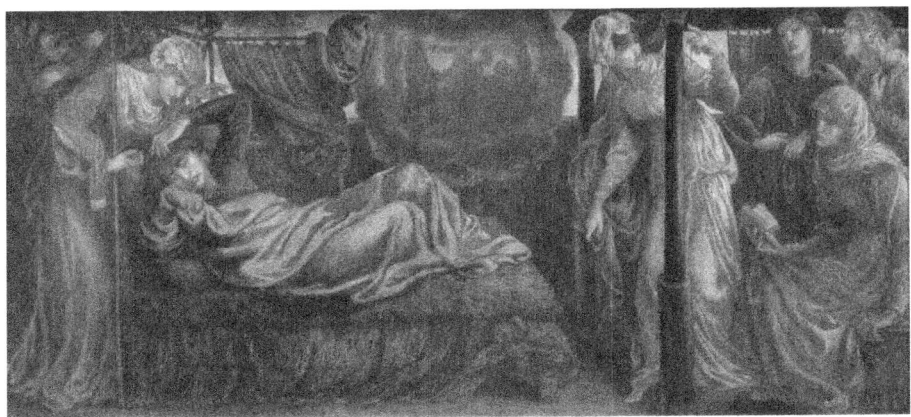

Figure 4-2: Rossetti's Dante's Dream on the Day of Death of Beatrice, 1880, *completed two years before his death. He had previously made other versions of this scene, going back to 1856. In a theme taken from Dante's poem 'La Vita Nuova', Dante has a vision in which he sees an angel in red bending forward to kiss the dying Beatrice, whom he has always loved. This particular version of the painting is taken from the Dundee Art Galleries and Museums Collection.*

REFERENCES for CHAPTER FOUR

Mendelson, W.B. : *Nepenthe's children: the History of the Discoveries of Medicines for Sleep and Anesthesia.* Pythagoras Press, 2020a.

https://www.amazon.com/dp/B08H4XDZBN

Mendelson W.B.: *The Curious History of Medicines in Psychiatry.* Pythagoras Press, 2020b.

https://www.amazon.com/dp/B083ZRMCW1

68

CHAPTER FIVE

EMILY DICKINSON, THE WOMAN IN WHITE

To write about Emily Dickinson is a very different experience than chronicling most of the other figures in this book. Though her life was relatively short, like those of Nikolai Gogol or Edgar Allan Poe, it had none of the exterior action, moving from city to city or job to job, and certainly none of the world travel of Melville or Darwin. She did not seek relief from distress in the Holy Land, as had Gogol and Melville, or the Scottish Highlands as had Darwin and Rossetti. Indeed, most of her life was spent in a single town—Amherst, Massachusetts—and in indeed in a single house. The action in her life was interior, and expressed in her letters and her poetry.

She was born in Amherst in 1830. Her father's family had come from England as part of the Puritan migrations of the early 1600s. Samuel Dickinson, her paternal grandfather, was a lawyer and founder of Amherst College, whose life was characterized by bursts of energy alternating with 'depression of spirits'; he was viewed as the black sheep of the family (McDermott, 2001). In 1813 he built a grand brick house, known as The Homestead, in Amherst. When in financial distress in 1828 he sold it, but in 1830 his lawyer son Edward bought back the western half of the house, and settled in with his wife, Emily Norcross Dickinson and their infant son Austin. Emily was born within the year, followed three years later by her sister Lavinia. It was the first brick house in town, located on Main Street; it had a barn and garden over an acre in size, which provided much of Emily's experience of nature. It was in her room at the Homestead that Lavinia later found her poems in a locked chest (just as Melville's *Billy Budd* was found by his granddaughter in a breadbox; Chapter one) and started the process of having them published.

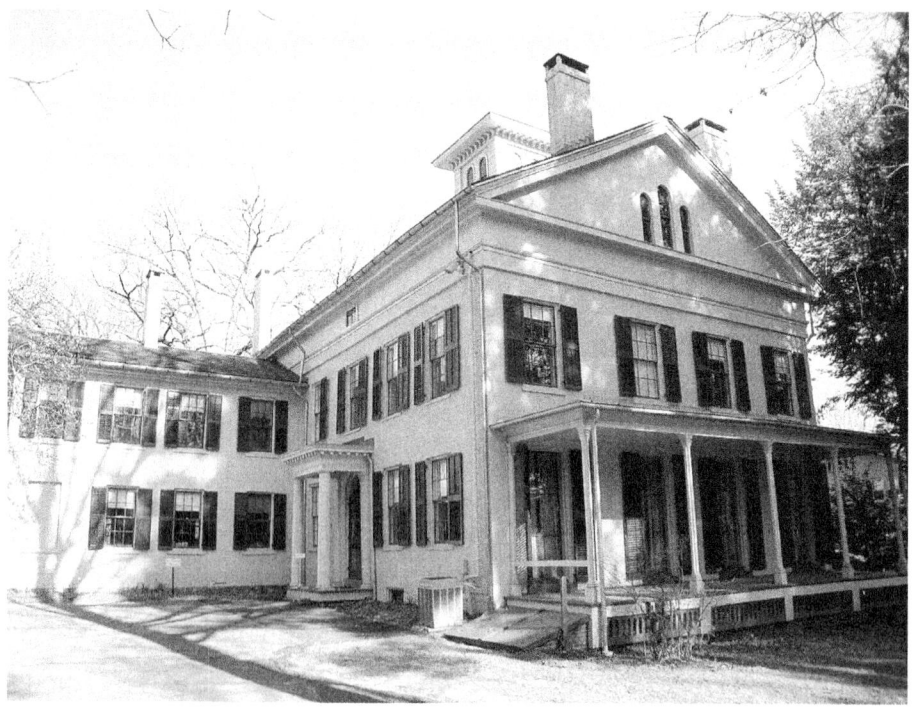

Figure 5-1: *The Homestead, in which Emily Dickinson was born and died, and lived all but about 15 years of her life. In 1855 she had a conservatory installed*

for her plant collections, just as Darwin built a heated greenhouse for his orchids. When she was in her 20s, her father built an adjacent house, The Evergreens, for her older brother Austin and his wife Susan, with whom Emily was very close. Both have been preserved by the Emily Dickinson Museum, and this photograph was taken in 2008.

Emily was described as well-behaved, though frail, and responded well to her father's enthusiasm for education. Her teachers recognized her skills with both the piano and composition. Though often away (he was a state legislator and later a U.S. congressman), Emily viewed him as warm and caring, feelings which she apparently believed she did not receive from her mother.

As Emily Norcross Dickinson is largely known through her daughter's eyes, it is difficult to get a full understanding of her. She came from nearby Monson, Massachusetts, and was well educated, having attended both Monson Academy and a boarding school in New Haven. After her marriage, which she seemed to enter into with some reluctance, she spent most of her time at The Homestead, where she was often alone because of her husband's travels. In her isolation she took care of the home, and seemed to get some consolation from gardening. Her relationship with the young Emily was distant, though in later years, when she was chronically ill and cared for by Emily, the two formed a closer bond.

In 1840 Emily entered Amherst Academy, previously a boys' school which had recently begun admitting girls. That same year the family moved to a more modest house, of which the children were fond, though the view was largely of Amherst's West Cemetery. In 1855 her father, then in a better financial position, bought back the entire Homestead, to which the family returned.

During her seven years at Amherst Academy, Emily was known as a good student, but due to vaguely described illnesses was frequently kept at home. To some degree these absences may have been related to what she referred to in her letters in adolescence as 'fixed melancholy' (Johnson and Ward, 1986). In 1844 her cousin Sophia Holland, to whom she felt very close, died of typhus. Emily's distress was so great, with thoughts of her own death, that her parents had her go to live with relatives in Boston. Two months later she returned with her melancholy seemingly improved. This was her first experience of losing a loved one, and thoughts of bereavement began to appear in her writings, primarily in the form of letters until her mid-20s. In a way Sophia Holland's death is reminiscent of Poe's loss of a woman toward whom he had romantic feelings when he was 15 (Chapter Three); in both instances, the experience was the beginning of the theme of loss which would affect their writing for years to come.

After her return to the Academy, she also made two acquaintances which were to alter her life. One was the young principal Leonard Humphrey, with whom she was friendly and who would later represent another loss in her life. The other was Susan Huntington Gilbert, a young woman who had been orphaned at an early age, now staying with her sister in Amherst. Emily and Susan became close friends, and later possibly something more. Jumping ahead some years, Susan later met Emily's older brother Austin in 1853 and married him in 1856. Many of Emily's letters to her are still available, and scholars argue to what degree the passionate closeness which Emily professed was literary metaphor or instead evidence of an actual romance.

After graduating from Amherst Academy in 1847, Emily attended Mount Holyoke Female Seminary (later Mount Holyoke College). She returned home after only 10 months for reasons which are not clear, perhaps unhappiness with its emphasis on religious devotion or health issues or homesickness. In the meantime, her thinking about religion and the place of humanity in the world continued to evolve. She had been brought up in a Calvinist family, which had strong beliefs that everything observable was based on immutable facts springing from a miraculous creation. As the nineteenth century progressed, the challenge from the more liberal views of Unitarianism led to a corresponding resurgence of Calvinist doctrine. Her reaction to this may have been part of the impetus for her to decline to make the public pronouncement of faith required for membership in her family's First Congregational Church, and to honor the sabbath at home rather than in church. Throughout her life she continued to have deep feelings about spirituality and immortality of the soul, though outside the context of organized Calvinist worship.

Dickinson's outward life in those years was one of attending to the house and social activities. During this time she met Benjamin Franklin Newton, a young attorney with a literary bent, who introduced her to the poetry of Wordsworth, Emerson and others. He was to become one of several older men she termed 'master' in her correspondence. In 1850, her former school principal Leonard Humphrey died unexpectedly. It was Dickinson's second loss, and it affected her deeply. In 1855 she and her mother traveled to Washington, where her father was serving as a congressman, and then visited family in Philadelphia. There she met a Presbyterian minister, Charles Wadsworth, to whom she became attached. Although they met in person only two more times, they developed a correspondence which went on until he passed away in 1882.

A few months after their return to Amherst, her mother became ill, and remained bedridden for most of the next three decades. The family had moved back into their original house, The Homestead, and the need to maintain this large dwelling and care for the mother occupied Emily and Lavinia. Emily began to withdraw more and more from social activities, though she continued active correspondence with friends, and with her sister-in-law Susan. The later 1850s were a difficult time, while the family was troubled by a lawsuit involving her mother's family and the distress of a railroad which had been supported by her father. There were bright spots as well. She became acquainted with Samuel Bowles, the owner of a newspaper based in Springfield, Massachusetts, and thus began a lengthy correspondence and the anonymous publication of a number of her poems. In these years she also wrote several of the 'Master Letters' mentioned earlier, passionate avowals of affection to an unknown gentleman who was thought to perhaps have been Bowles, though later research suggested that some were written before they were acquainted.

In 1858 Dickinson withdrew socially even more, and entered what were to be her most productive years. She assembled her earlier poems into fascicles (notebooks of pages sewn together), and wrote perhaps 800 more by 1865. As we will discuss later, in the first few years there appears to be a pattern of decreased writing in winter compared to summer months, raising speculation about a possible role of seasonal affective disorder (McDermott, 2001).

In the fall of 1861 she entered a difficult period she was later to refer to as the 'terror'. It has never been fully explained, but may have involved disappointment at the lack of romantic reciprocation from the never-identified 'Master', Samuel Bowles' ill health, or the perceived emotional withdrawal by Susan who was having her first child (Habegger, 2001). It is likely that she began to feel abandoned and alone, but turned her distress into a kind of defiance and source of strength. In an often-quoted 1862 poem she wrote:

The Zeroes—taught us—Phosphorous—

We learned to like the Fire

By playing Glaciers—when a Boy—

And Tinder—guessed—by power

Of Opposite—to balance Odd—

If White—a Red—must be!

Paralysis—our Primer—dumb—

Unto Vitality!

(Wikisource, 2013)

Phosphorus matches had become popular since their introduction in the 1820s, and were made safer with the less toxic red phosphorus in 1855. For Dickinson, they apparently emblemized the ability of fire to blaze suddenly even in cold conditions; by implication, coldness can suddenly turn to vitality and creativity. It certainly was a period in which her own creativity—and ambition as well—were sparked.

In April 1862 she had seen an article by the literary critic Thomas Wentworth Higginson giving advice to new authors. It has been speculated that she may have been feeling frustrated at not having outlets to let the world see her poetry. She wrote Higginson describing her situation, and he sent back supportive letters which she later said had saved her life during this difficult time. Dickinson associated the end of the 'terror' with the beginning of a period of even greater productivity, and indeed from 1862 to 1865 she created more than half of her lifetime work. Some of her poems were inspired by the suffering caused by the Civil War, while others were more optimistic, emphasizing a sense of growing self-reliance and pride in skillful creativity. By 1865 her work was interrupted by eye difficulties requiring trips to see doctors in Boston, and by 1866 her output declined.

It was a difficult time for Dickinson. Their family maid who had helped for a decade left, and was not replaced until 1869. During this time many more household duties fell on her shoulders, and in this period she also lost her pet dog who had been her companion since the early 1850s. She became even more withdrawn, rarely leaving the house. On those occasions in which she did, she wore light colored clothing, and became known in the neighborhood as 'the woman in white'. On the rare occasions when visitors would appear, she would not see them in person, but rather would talk from behind a door. What little social life she had was conducted primarily through letters and small gifts. Rather than see the neighborhood children in person, she would send down baskets of gingerbread from her second story window. The one notable exception to her withdrawal was her relationship with Otis Phillips Lord, a judge with whom she shared literary thoughts, and whose interest may have become more romantic a few years later after his wife passed away.

In these years Dickinson's view of religion and man's place in the world continued to evolve as well. Darwin's publication of *On the Origin of Species* in 1859 (Chapter six) had led to widespread debate challenging the Calvinist notion that the world was based on immutable facts, among which was that mankind was created by a miracle and thus quite apart from the rest of nature. Darwin pictured a very different kind of world, which was constantly, though slowly, changing, with continents rising and mountains appearing across geological time, and with a similar fluid process leading to the evolving of species. Dickinson, like Darwin, was influenced by the death of loved ones as well seeing the seeming brutality of nature in the lives of small creatures in their gardens and woods. These experiences made it easier to understand human beings as not being exceptional in their creation, but rather part of the natural world. Dickinson mentioned Darwin several times in her letters (Mondello, 2020) and become more comfortable with the notion that the world was not immutably fixed, but in a state of fluidity.

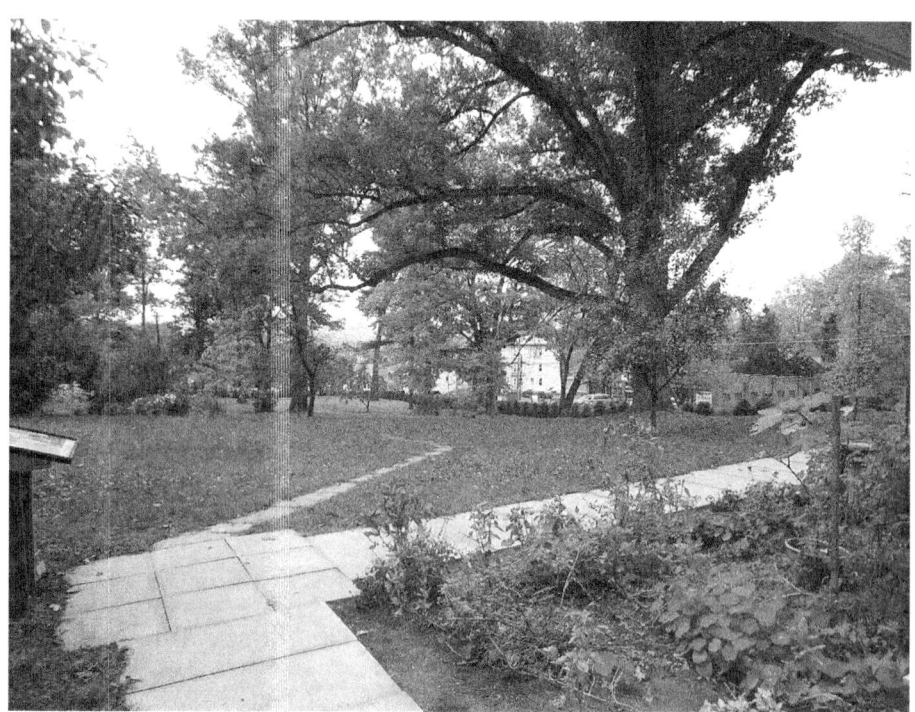

Figure 5-2: *View of the back yard of The Homestead, as maintained by the Emily Dickinson Museum, in a photograph taken in 2013.*

In 1874 Dickinson's father died of a stroke while on a trip to Boston. The funeral took place in the front room of their home, but she did not attend; instead, she listened from behind her upstairs bedroom door. The following year a stroke left her mother partially paralyzed and affected her memory. Dickinson's writing declined to about 35 poems a year as she dealt with loss and her caretaking responsibilities.

The year 1882 was notable for both the death of her mother, and also a family complication: her brother Austin had begun a rather public affair with Mabel Loomis Todd, the wife of an astronomy professor at Amherst, and to some degree he withdrew from his closeness with the rest of the family. The following year her nephew, Austin's son Gilbert, to whom she was particularly attached, died, followed over the next decade by her friends Samuel Bowles, Charles Wadsworth, and Otis Phillips Lord. Isolated and seeing almost no one, her health deteriorated. By late 1885 she was frail and mostly stayed in bed; she passed away, from what at the time was thought to be Bright's disease (chronic nephritis) in May 1886. She was interred in a white coffin with flowers she had chosen, a lady slipper orchid, heliotrope and violets.

Later, her sister Lavinia found her papers, including correspondence and some 1700 poems. Lavinia honored Emily's wish to burn her letters, but had been left with no clear instructions about the poetry.

Lavinia wanted to see them published, and turned them over, perhaps unwisely, to both Austin's wife Susan as well as his lover Mabel Loomis Todd. A small volume, heavily edited by Todd and Thomas Wentworth Higginson, appeared in 1890, followed by other small collections, but the inevitable squabble between the two women and then their children delayed the publication of the complete works for several decades. Even in the early years the quality and freshness of the poems was recognized by luminaries such as William Dean Howells. Growing critical recognition, and then the later notoriety of having competing volumes issued by the daughters of Susan and Mabel continued to spark public interest. Many more editions appeared in the early 20th century, but it was not until the 1950's that the first complete and scholarly collections became available.

* * *

Emily Dickinson's quiet, secluded life has been viewed many different ways over the years. Since the first complete volumes appeared in the 1950s, it is not surprising that many analyses of that time had a psychoanalytic bent, often emphasizing the effects of a domineering father, a cold mother and an 'ambiguous sexuality'. It was often suggested that as a result of a poor relationship with her mother she felt unloved, and was hesitant to grow into a woman's role lest she come to resemble her.

Psychoanalytic interpretations later came under criticism for emphasizing sexuality at the cost of neglecting other influences including social standards, women's roles both in college and the community, the religious movements of the time, and authors she admired such as Charlotte Brontë and Elizabeth Browning (Tanner, 1987). In the next few decades the suggestion was made that seclusion was a reasonable and consciously adopted lifestyle which made her work possible. Psychiatrist John McDermott, in an analysis of her letters, suggested that at age 24 she had an episode which met formal criteria for a panic attack, and the beginning of agoraphobia (McDermott, 2000). In a later study he argued that during the first half of her most productive years, 1858-1865, the number of poems she wrote was much greater in the spring and summer compared to fall and winter, suggesting that she suffered from seasonal affective disorder (McDermott, 2001). This process was interrupted by the emotional upset we described earlier, which she termed the 'terror'. The end of the terror led to the beginning of an even more remarkably productive four years, which he noted might be consistent with bipolar II disorder (see Addendum).

Certainly, Dickinson left much evidence of being very sensitive to the seasons, and on numerous occasions she likened the winter months to death. One issue militating against the interpretation that her productivity in the years 1862-1865 was primarily related to hypomania is the very long duration; in data developed more recently than the McDermott (2001) study, about three-quarters of hypomanic episodes in bipolar II disorder were reported to be for less than four weeks (Benzazzi and Akiskal, 2006). There are, of course, alternative or additional interpretations to her remarkable increase in productivity after the 'terror'. One would be that she now had the support of Thomas Wentworth Higginson, who as we noted she later credited with saving her life. Another would be that her new productivity was a response to having been so focused on death; indeed, she likened her new work to being like the boy who sings as he passes a graveyard. Viewed in this way, her output in those years might reflect the maturing and blossoming of a creative response to a period of depression.

Two decades later, when she was 53, Dickinson's physician believed that she suffered from 'nervous prostration'. At the time this was considered a form of neurasthenia manifested as fatigue, anxiety and depressed mood (Beard, 1869). Aside from this we know little of how her condition was viewed at the time. We do know that her life was marked by a number of deaths of persons to whom she was close, beginning with her cousin when she was 14, and that her response was so great that the family felt the need to send her away to live with relatives in Boston. Both her letters and poetry dwell on thoughts of loss, of which she experienced many.

In more recent years it has been recognized that about 10-20 percent of bereaved persons develop what was first called 'complicated grief' and is now formalized as 'prolonged grief disorder'. Persons with this condition continue to grieve more than a year after the event, and manifest many of the symptoms of depression, though with some subtle differences. Their self-derogatory thoughts, for instance, do not reflect an overall sense of worthlessness, but rather are oriented to belief in their having failed the loved one, and thoughts of death center on the lost loved one and the notion of joining them (Parkes, 2020). Whether this might fit Emily Dickinson, or whether this is an over-medicalization of a reaction to a universal human experience, is a specific case of an issue being debated for society at large. What we can say is that she was very sensitive to the loss of important figures, either through death or perceived withdrawal of affection. We can speculate whether this inhibited her work or whether instead she was able to transform these thoughts creatively into poetry. Like many of the other figures in this book such as Herman Melville and Nikolai Gogol, the life of the writer has been as rich a source of fascination and supposition as the writings themselves.

REFERENCES for CHAPTER FIVE

Beard, G.M.: Neurasthenia or nervous exhaustion. Boston Med. Surgical J. 3: 217-220, 1869.

https://scholar.google.com/scholar?hl=en&q=Beard+GM%3A+Neurasthenia+or+nervous+exhaustion.+Boston+Med+Surgical+J+1869%3B+3%3A217–220

Benazzi, F. and Akiskal, H.: The duration of hypomania in bipolar-II disorder in private practice: methodology and validation. J. Affect. Disord. 96: 189-196, 2006.

https://pubmed.ncbi.nlm.nih.gov/16427136/

Feist, G.J.: A meta-analysis of personality in scientific and artistic creativity. Pers. Soc. Psychol. Rev. 2:: 290-309, 1998.

https://pubmed.ncbi.nlm.nih.gov/15647135/

Habegger, A.: *My wars are laid away in books: the life of Emily Dickinson.* Random House, 2001.

https://www.amazon.com/Wars-Are-Laid-Away-Books-ebook/dp/B000FC1JGM

Johnson, T.H. and Ward, T. (eds.): *The letters of Emily Dickinson.* The Belknap Press of Harvard University Press, Cambridge, 1986.

McDermott, J.F.: Emily Dickinson's 'nervous prostration' and its possible relationship to her work. The Emily Dickinson Journal 9: 71-86, 2000).

https://muse.jhu.edu/article/11140

McDermott, J.F.: Emily Dickinson revisited: a study of periodicity in her work. Am. J. Psychiatry online May 1, 2001.

https://ajp.psychiatryonline.org/doi/10.1176/appi.ajp.158.5.686

Mondello, K.: "Of toads and men": brutal kinship in Emily Dickinson and Charles Darwin. J. Literature and Science. 13: 1-19, 2020.

Parkes, C.M.: Complicated grief in the DSM-5: problems and solutions. Arch. Psychiatr. Ment. Health 4: 48-51, 2020.

https://www.heighpubs.org/hjcap/apmh-aid1019.php Accessed April 27, 2021.

Tanner, S.L.: Emily Dickinson and the psychoanalyst. Estudos Germanicos 8:6, December 1987.

https://www.researchgate.net/publication/287930004_Emily_Dickinson_and_the_psychoanalyst

Wikisource: The zeroes—taught us—phosphorus—. Wikisource, last edited March 1, 2013. Available under the Creative Commons Attribution-ShareAlike License.

https://en.wikisource.org/wiki/The_Zeroes_—_taught_us_—_Phosphorous_—

CHAPTER SIX

CHARLES DARWIN, ILLNESS AND THE DISTRACTIONS OF SOCIETY

Charles Darwin produced neither fiction nor poetry, but he was a remarkably productive writer who creatively developed the concept of evolution by natural selection, thus profoundly altering the course of biological thinking for generations. Interestingly, his life's work may have been influenced by the poetry of his grandfather, Erasmus Darwin, who in 'The Temple of Nature' had speculated about what came to be known as evolution and the origins of mankind (Simon, 2019). As we described in the Introduction, Charles also made many drawings of his specimens, worked with artists to make others, and was one of the first to use photographic illustrations. As we will see in this chapter, like Dickinson he lived his later life in seclusion from which his prodigious works emerged, though unlike Dickinson his thoughts were recognized—and became a subject of controversy— during his lifetime.

Born in 1809 in Shropshire, he was the son of Robert Darwin, a wealthy doctor and financier, and his wife Susanna, a member of the

Wedgwood family famous for manufacturing fine porcelain and china. When he was eight, his mother developed abdominal pains and died shortly thereafter, and he was raised largely by his older sisters. He was a generally healthy and vigorous teen whose main enthusiasm was in hunting and shooting, though he was troubled occasionally by stomach upsets at breakfast and outbreaks of boils. His father, worried about his seeming lack of serious interests, enrolled him at age 16 in the medical school at Edinburgh University. He quickly lost interest in medicine, apparently distressed by witnessing surgery, but was stimulated by teachers into studying natural sciences, particularly marine invertebrates. His father began to believe that an education as an Anglican clergyman might provide more structure to his life, and transferred him to Christ's College, Cambridge. There Charles was able to enjoy the pastimes of young gentlemen, but also came under the influence of traditionally trained naturalists, accompanying one on a trip to study the geology of Wales. After graduating in 1831, one of his botany teachers suggested that he join a voyage on the *HMS Beagle* to the southern tip of South America. Rather than serve in the crew, he enthusiastically paid his own way as a companion to the aristocratic captain who desired time with someone of his own class and upbringing.

Darwin arrived in Plymouth in October 1831, excited but also anxious about leaving his family and the world he knew. The beginning of his adventure was not propitious; the *Beagle* set out twice unsuccessfully, forced back by gales, and was delayed again after excessive carousing at Christmastime. 'These two months at Plymouth were the most miserable which I ever spent', he later wrote. 'I was also troubled with palpitation and pain about the heart, and like many a young ignorant man, especially one with a smattering of medical knowledge, was convinced that I had heart disease. I did not consult any doctor, as I fully expected to hear the verdict that I was not fit for the voyage, and I was resolved to go at all hazards.' (F. Darwin, 1887).

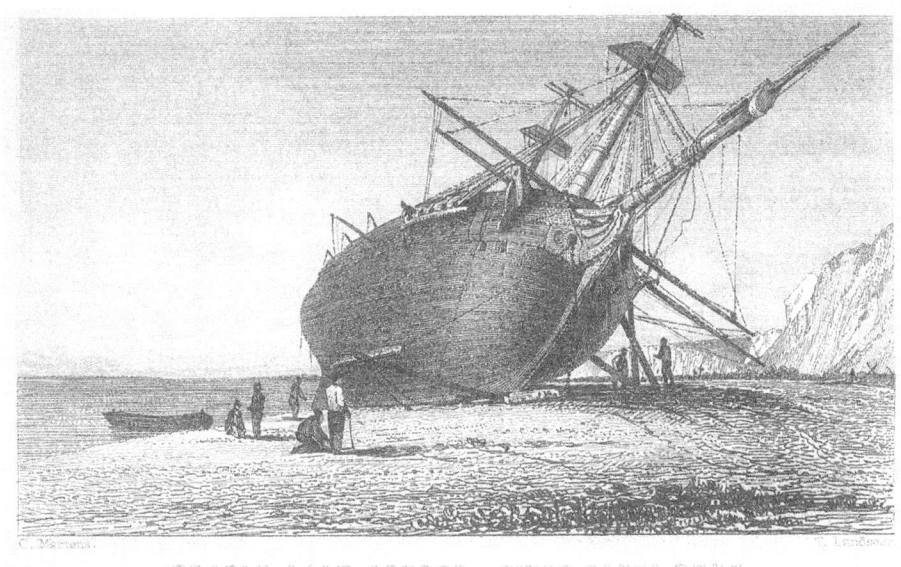

Figure 6-1: HMS Beagle *undergoing repairs by the Santa Cruz River, Argentina, 1839. It was a brig-sloop originally with 10 guns, built by the Royal Navy in 1820. Its length was 90.3 ft., with a beam of 24.5 ft. During the coronation ceremonies for King George IV it traveled up the Thames and was the first rigged warship to pass through the old London Bridge. It later sailed on three survey expeditions, the second of which was described in Darwin's journal, and published as* The Voyage of the Beagle.

Finally on December 27, 1831 the *Beagle* successfully began its five year voyage. It was a trying time for Darwin's health. In addition to persistent seasickness, he suffered from fevers, boils, heat stroke, food poisoning, and inflammation of the knee and arm (Cohen and Mackowiak, 2013; Colp, 1977). Despite these difficulties his studies were prodigious. While at sea he dragged nets in the water and reported on plankton. As a self-funded traveler, he had a great deal of freedom, and managed to spend all but 18 months on land (Brown and Neve, 1989), while the Beagle continued its surveying work. In the Cape Verde Islands he was fascinated with the bands of oysters embedded in the cliffs, and speculated about the shifts in the landscape across time. He marveled at the rain forests of Brazil, and in Patagonia discovered the fossilized bones of huge ancient mammals. In the Andes he made watercolors of rock formations (Zimmer, 2009), and found seashells and fossilized seashore vegetation. He had been heavily influenced by the Scottish geologist Charles Lyell, who argued that the earth was created by natural processes which could still be observed, and he was fascinated with the notion of the rise and fall of the land across geologic time. In the Galapagos he noted how mockingbirds and finches had different characteristics on each island. He collected thousands of specimens of fossils, insects, plants, birds, eggs and nests, many of which he shipped back to England along the way. He had begun the voyage as a 22-year-old planning to become a clergyman, who was indulging his interest in biology and geology; he returned as a seasoned scientist with a growing reputation from the materials he had sent ahead (American Museum of Natural History, 2021). He brought back extensive journals and notebooks filled with materials and questions which would last him a lifetime.

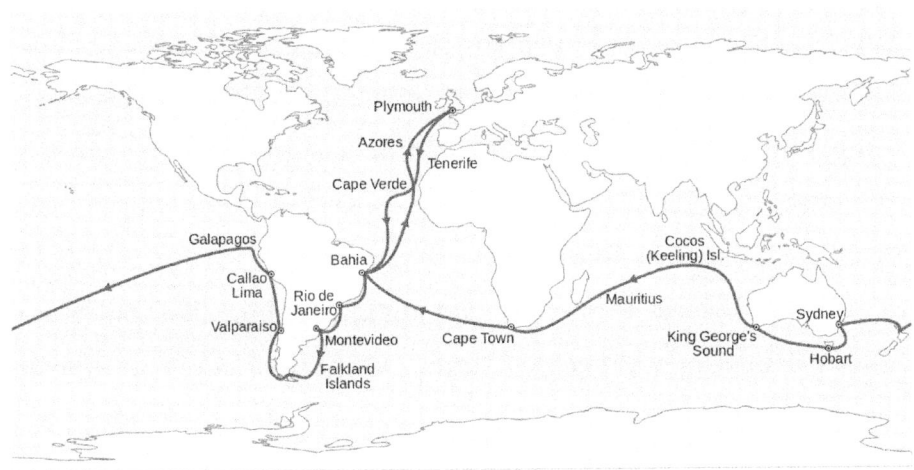

Figure 6-2: *Map of the round-the-world voyage of* HMS Beagle. *It embarked on December 27, 1831, for what was originally planned to be a two year voyage, but ended up taking almost five years. During this time Darwin kept a diary which grew to 770 pages, which became the basis of his 1839 book popularly known as* The Voyage of the Beagle. *Although it contained some inklings of his growing thoughts on natural selection, elaborated more in a later 1845 edition, his formal theory of evolution did not come to fruition until the publication of* On the Origin of Species *two decades later.*

Darwin began working in London in March 1837, writing and categorizing his specimens, and discussing his findings with Charles Lyell and other scholars. In 1837 he presented his first paper to the Geological Society, indicating that the coastline of Chile was rising. Aided by investments from his father as well as government funding, he hired artists to illustrate his specimens, which he published in *Zoology of the Voyage of HMS Beagle (1838-1843).*

Initially Darwin's health seemed good, but after about 18 months he developed abdominal pain with frequent nausea and vomiting (often after every meal), which would afflict him for many years to come. Like Gogol (Chapter two), as a young man he developed a variety of symptoms which were never well explained. Darwin complained of palpitations, insomnia, numbness in his fingers, tremor and a buzzing sound inside his head (Cohen and Mackowiak, 2013). He recognized that these were associated with times of stress; in 1838 he traveled to the Scottish Highlands for relief, but found himself studying the geology, much as he had done during his voyage on the *Beagle*. At one point he found what he believed was evidence of beaches which over eons had risen into the mountains, as he had in Chile, but this time was later forced to acknowledge that instead they were the remains of ancient lakes (Barlow, 1958a). He returned briefly refreshed. In the ensuing months he proposed to his first cousin, Emma Wedgwood, and they were married in January 1839. He continued to apply himself to his work, though his various symptoms soon reappeared.

By 1842 he had finished an outline of what would later grow into *On the Origin of Species*, and sought solitude in a former parsonage in the small village of Downe, in Kent. There he led a very organized life, his days arranged with precision into scheduled times for study, walking and resting. He avoided scientific meetings and their resultant stress whenever possible. He continued to worry about the condemnation with which his ideas were likely to be found be the clergy-dominated thinking of the time. He was also very much aware that the notion of 'transmutation' (which anticipated evolution) promulgated by his poet/physician grandfather Erasmus Darwin had led to criticism and sometimes vilification. These were difficult times for him, particularly with the death by typhoid of his oldest daughter Annie in 1851, which led him to question his religious beliefs. His many physical symptoms continued, and he sought relief at spas and with unusual treatments such as affixing batteries to his abdomen.

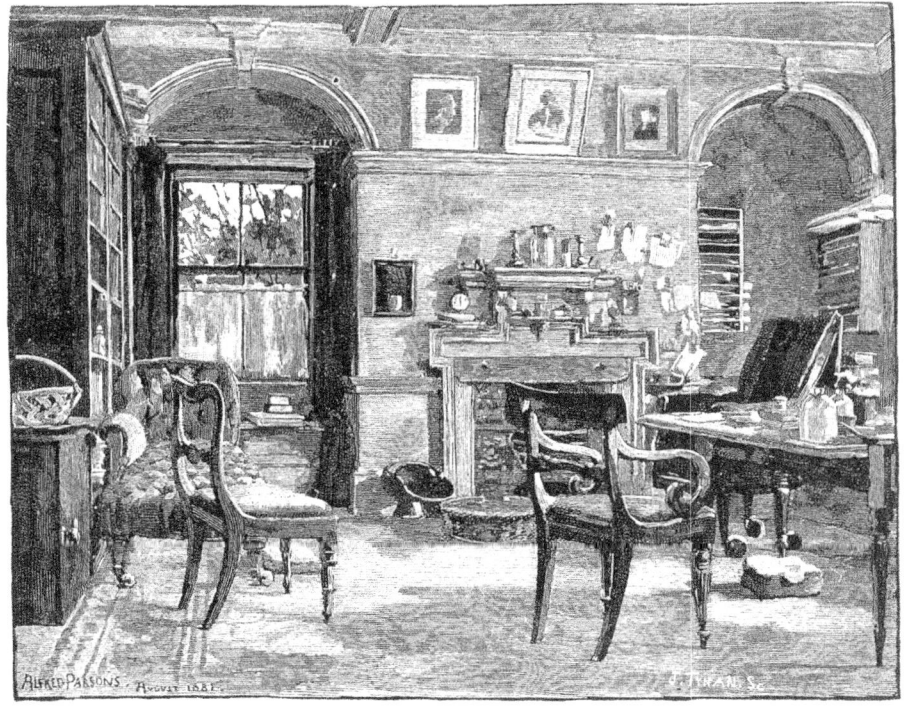

DARWIN'S STUDY.

Figure 6-3: *Darwin's study in Downe, Kent, as depicted* in Charles Darwin: His Life and Work *by Charles Frederick Holder, 1891. Darwin moved into this former parsonage in 1842 and lived primarily there until his death in 1882. Over the years he added many features, including a heated greenhouse for his studies of orchid fertilization, complete with a tunnel to allow entry of bees.*

By the 1850s, however, the world was also changing. In the 1830s when Darwin was first formulating his ideas about how new species might develop, the Anglican church, which viewed the origins of the world and man as resulting from miracles, was dominant. As time went on it began to be challenged by radical nonconformists who were more open to the idea of the transmutation of species. Two decades later, science and society at large were becoming more secular, as epitomized by the rise in prominence of the biologist Thomas Henry Huxley, and the philosopher Herbert Spencer. After talks with Huxley and the famed botanist Joseph Dalton Hooker, Darwin began organizing and writing his ideas going back over two decades in a work he tentatively entitled *Natural Selection.* From notions that the very earth changed, with coastlines rising and falling over time, grew the idea that species of living creatures might also change into new forms.

Despite the stress of finding that his tenth child, Charles Waring Darwin, was developmentally disabled, he continued to work, and by 1858 had a substantial manuscript in hand. It was then that he received a professional shock: Alfred Russel Wallace, a naturalist working in the Dutch East Indies, sent him an essay outlining ideas about natural selection that closely mirrored his own. Greatly distressed, Darwin consulted Lyell and Hooker, who formulated a plan: they would present the work of both men jointly at a scientific meeting in July 1858. Darwin, himself, dealing with the recent death from scarlet fever of his son, was unable to attend. He continued working frantically on his manuscript. When the book, now entitled *On the Origin of Species',* came out in November 1859, the fifty-year-old Darwin was away at a spa in a remote area of Yorkshire.

The years following publication of his master work were marked by both controversy but also support from colleagues such as Huxley. Though he avoided public meetings, Darwin continued to update his views in six editions of the book, and gathered further evidence from studies of domestic plants and animals. He also continued to write copiously in his health diary, precisely recording his symptoms and the status of his bodily processes. He worried that his mother's death during his childhood suggested that he and his children might have inherited some form of constitutional weakness. He consulted a large assortment of physicians, who were unable to find specific physical signs behind his symptoms, and they gave him a range of diagnoses including hypochondriasis, hyperventilation, allergies and gout. He began to have crying spells while complaining of 'lumbago' and 'rheumatism', as well as skin eruptions (Colp, 1977; Cohen and Mackowiak, 2013). Sometimes he seemed unable to speak or appeared to have partial paralysis or memory loss (Hayman, 2013; Jones, 1867). He received a wide range of treatments including bismuth, arsenic, strychnine, calomel (mercury), mineral acids, codeine, and plant extracts. None seemed to help aside from cold water baths, which seemed to briefly ease his gastric complaints.

I think

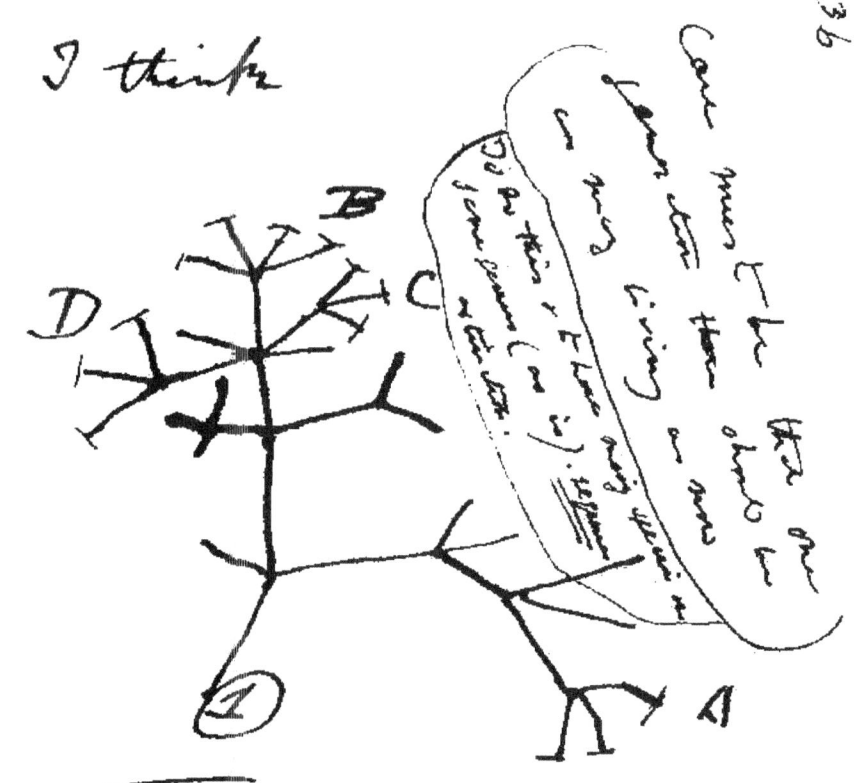

Then between A. & B. immens
gap of relation. C & B. the
finest gradation, B & D
rather greater distinction
Then genera would be
formed. — bearing relation

Figure 6-4: *Darwin's first drawing depicting an evolutionary tree, which* *appeared in his* First Notebook on Transmutation of Species *in 1837. His* *handwriting has been interpreted to read: "I think case must be that one* *generation should have as many living as now. To do this and to have as many* *species in same genus (as is) requires extinction. Thus between A + B the* *immense gap of relation. C + B the finest gradation. B+D rather greater* *distinction. Thus genera would be formed. Bearing relation"* (next page begins) *"to ancient types with several extinct forms"* (From user 'fileunderwater' at https://biology.stackexchange.com/questions/46481 /darwins-first-sketch-of-a-phylogenetic-tree, accessed on April 26, 2021.)

In later years, Darwin had mixed feelings about his illnesses. Though he had had often regretted periods in which he felt too sick to work, he also noted 'Even ill-health, though it has annihilated several years of my life, has saved me from the distractions of society and amusement.' (Barlow, 1958b). He continued to work, and in 1872, at age 63, came out with *The Expression of the Emotions in Man and Animals*, one of the first books to include photographs (Zimmer, 1009). Many of his symptoms seemed less severe in older age. One interpretation was that he was engaged in less controversial subjects (Kalb, 2016), such as his last book at age 71, *The Formation of Vegetable Mould Through the Action of Earthworms*. (One is reminded of the retired Sherlock Holmes devoting himself to beekeeping.) Another way of looking at it is that he was being true to his longstanding beliefs that over the ages small incremental actions could produce profound effects. In this case, he was arguing that even the lowly earthworm, given geological time, could alter the very topography of the earth. It also had personal meaning to him, as he contemplated death and burial in the soil, with acceptance and comments that he was ready. By now he was having anginal symptoms, and for the first time in his life, doctors were able to point to active heart disease as a physical counterpart to his symptoms (Cohen and Mackowiak, 2013). He passed away peacefully in 1882, expressing kind words and thanks to his wife and children. Though he had thought he would be buried in the local churchyard, his friends and colleagues successfully petitioned for him to be laid to rest in an honored place at Westminster Abbey.

* * *

There has been ongoing fascination with Darwin's health. He was examined and treated by some of the most respected physicians of his day, who left a legacy of a wide range of diagnoses, and subsequently over the years various writers have suggested at least 40 more (Colp, 2008). Among these were neurasthenia, cyclical vomiting syndrome, Crohn's disease, peptic ulcer, brucellosis, arsenic poisoning, Meniere's disease, and many others. In a sense, Darwin became a kind of mirror, in which prominent physicians have seen reflections of their specialties. Saul Adler, an Israeli tropical medicine specialist, suggested that he suffered from Chagas disease (American trypanosomiasis), resulting from parasites transmitted by insect bites in South America (Adler, 1959). Barry Marshall, the Nobel Prize winner who had discovered *Helicobacter pylori* bacteria which can cause peptic ulcer disease, proposed that this was the source of Darwin's distress (Marshall, 2009). John Hayman, an Australian pathologist, argued that Darwin's symptoms as well as his family history, might be due to MELAS syndrome, a maternally inherited mitochondrial DNA disorder (Hayman, 2013).

A similar process has taken place in psychiatry. In the years in which psychoanalysis was a dominant movement in European psychiatry, John Bowlby suggested that Darwin's adult symptoms resulted from the experience of his mother's sudden death when he was eight years old (Bowlby, 1965). Other psychodynamic theories have been that his symptoms resulted from Oedipal jealousy of his father, or anger toward his wife Emma. An idea going back to his original physicians was that he suffered from hypochondriasis, and it has been argued by Cohen and Mackowiak (2103) and others that he met most of the modern criteria for the diagnosis (now considered to be one of the somatic symptom disorders). He differed from many typical patients, however, in that he did not respond to reassurance with frustration, but rather with gratitude, and he recognized that anxiety might play a role in his condition (Cohen and Mackowiak, 2013). His palpitations, chest discomfort, fear that he might be dying, and other symptoms have led Barloon and Noyes (1997) and others to make a strong case that he suffered from panic disorder with agoraphobia.

Other psychiatric diagnoses may arise as, inevitably, future generations will continue to puzzle over Darwin's health. What we can say is that he suffered greatly for most of his adult life, and a panoply of doctors, including some of the most well-known in their time, were unable to point to clear physical conditions until heart disease was recognized in his 70s. It is also possible that he had unrecognized medical illnesses which were exacerbated by anxiety. The remarkable feature of Darwin's health is that although it compromised his social functioning, he was able to work creatively for decades, and put together a new view of mankind which continues to influence our thinking to this day.

REFERENCES for CHAPTER SIX

Adler, S.: Darwin's illness. Nature 184:1102-1103, 1959.

American Museum of Natural History: A trip around the world. (Part of the Darwin exhibition.) Accessed April 8, 2021.
https://www.amnh.org/exhibitions/darwin/a-trip-around-the-world

Barloon, T.J. and Noyes, R. Jr.: Charles Darwin and Panic Disorder. JAMA 277: 138-141, 1997.
https://pubmed.ncbi.nlm.nih.gov/8990339/

Barlow, Nora, ed. (1958a) *The autobiography of Charles Darwin 1809-1882.* Collins, London. In Darwin Online, accessed April 9, 2021.
http://darwin-online.org.uk/content/frameset?viewtype=text&itemID=F1497&pageseq=86

Barlow, Nora, ed. (1958b) *The autobiography of Charles Darwin 1809-1882.* Collins, London. In Darwin Online, accessed April 11, 2021.

http://darwin-online.org.uk/content/frameset?viewtype=text&itemID=F1497&pageseq=150

Bowlby, J.: Darwin's health. Brit. Med. J., April 10, 1965, p. 999. https://www.ncbi.nlm.nih.gov/pmc/articles/PMC2165689/pdf/brmedj02389-0089c.pdf

Browne, E.J. and Neve, M.: 'Introduction' in Darwin, C.: *Voyage of the Beagle: Charles Darwin's journal of researches.* Penguin Books, London, 1989.

Colp, R. Jr.: *To be an invalid. The illness of Charles Darwin.* University of Chicago Press, Chicago, 1977.

Colp, R. Jr.: *Darwin's illness.* University Press of Florida, Gainseville, Florida, 2008.

Darwin, F. (ed.): *The life and letters of Charles Darwin, including an autobiographical chapter, Volume 1.* John Murray, London, 1887.

Hayman, J.: Charles Darwin's mitochondria. Genetics 194: 21-25, 2013. https://www.ncbi.nlm.nih.gov/pmc/articles/PMC3632469/

Kalb, C.: Evolution and angst: Charles Darwin was a worrier. Scientific American, February 11, 2016. Accessed April 11, 2021.

https://www.scientificamerican.com/article/evolution-and-angst-charles-darwin-was-a-worrier-excerpt/

Jones, H.B., 1867: Letter 5639—Jones, H.B. to Darwin, Emma, in *Darwin Correspondence Project Database.*
http://www.darwinproject.ac.uk/entry-5639/ Accessed December 9, 2010.

Marshall, B.: Darwin's illness was Helicobacter pylori. What I know and what I think I know. Accessed April 9, 2021.
http://barryjmarshall.blogspot.com/2009/02/darwins-illness-was-helicobacter-pylori.html

Simon, E.: How Erasmus Darwin's poetry prophesied evolutionary theory. Aeon.com, May 29, 2019.
https://aeon.co/ideas/how-erasmus-darwins-poetry-prophesied-evolutionary-theory

Zimmer, C.: Drawing from Darwin. Nature 458: 705, 2009.
https://www.nature.com/articles/458705a

CLOSING COMMENTS

We've seen, then, the stories of six individuals living around the same time—writers, poets, an artist, and a scientist highly influenced by the arts—who produced remarkably creative work while living very troubled lives. These short biographies have been designed to capture what it was like for them to be in the midst of both inner turmoil and remarkable creativity. The goal has been to give a sense that such struggles did not prevent them—some would say may have even aided them—in leaving a legacy in art and science that move us all these years later.

The Addendum which follows is for those who would like to pursue this subject in more detail. The economist Paul Krugman, who writes opinion pieces for the *New York Times*, has the delightful policy of letting his letting readers know in advance when a particular article will be more academic and technical by adding the phrases 'Wonkish' or 'Wonking out' following the title, and this Addendum might carry that notice. The first part describes studies of mental illness and creativity. The second focuses on the life of Abraham Lincoln, suggesting that the coexistence of mental illness, in his case severe depression, and the achievement of greatness is not confined to the arts.

ADDENDUM

Part 1

Creativity and mental illness

Though the notion that artists are often inflicted with madness goes back to ancient times, it was not until the 1950's and 1960's that Western scholars began systematic studies to explore the process of creativity. Frank Barron, one of the leaders of this new movement at the University of California, Berkeley, summarized the results of his work by saying that creative individuals are 'at once both naïve and knowledgeable, destructive and constructive, occasionally crazier yet adamantly saner' than most people (Barron, 1963). In the years that followed, one of the most influential studies was done in 1987 by Nancy Andreasen, who in addition to practicing psychiatry has a PhD in English literature. Though the study was of small size (30 creative writers at the Iowa Writers' Workshop and matched non-writers), it was unusual in that rather than examining scores on rating scales, it was based on actual diagnoses derived from psychiatric interviews (Andreasen, 1987). She found that writers were much more likely to have diagnosable illnesses, especially mood disorders (80 percent, including 37 percent depression and 43 percent bipolar disorder) compared to the non-writers (30 percent). A similar pattern was found in their families as well. Both groups were of above average intelligence, and differed only in that writers did better on a measure of vocabulary; this was taken to imply that intelligence *per se* and creativity are in some senses independent.

Many subsequent studies continued to find high rates of mood disorders or related symptoms in creative people; the Johns Hopkins psychologist Kay Redfield Jamison, for instance, found that in a group of prizewinning British writers and artists, 38 percent had been treated for mood disorders (Jamison, 1989). While not all of the more recent studies have found this kind of association (Pavrita et al., 2007), many have, including reports of higher rates of neuroticism in artists (Feist, 1998),mood disorder symptoms in creative individuals (Taylor, 2017), and high vulnerability to anxiety and depressive symptoms in visual artists (Ivcevic et al., 2020a). Andreasen (2008), writing two decades after her landmark study, concluded that most data suggest a higher rate of mood disorders in writers, but also recognized the limitations of such studies, including the problem of selecting appropriate comparison groups and the ongoing difficulty in defining creativity.

What are mood disorders?

Mood disorders refer to several common illnesses which primarily affect the emotions. They differ from the normal fluctuations in mood which everyone experiences in severity and duration, as well as their effect on functioning. Among them are:

Major depression: characterized by symptoms including negative mood, fatigue, decreased interest or feelings of pleasure, difficulty concentrating or focusing, insomnia, feelings of worthlessness or hopelessness, or thoughts of suicide, lasting at least two weeks. Another form of depression (dysthymia) may have less dramatic symptoms and last for prolonged periods (over two years). Another, sometimes referred to as 'minor depression' appears inside the category of 'Other specified depressive disorder' and refers to the presence of depressive symptoms which do not meet the full criteria of major depression.

Bipolar disorder: Periods of depression alternate with manic episodes of increased energy, elevated mood, irritability, disconnected or rapidly changing thoughts, and grandiosity, going on for at least a week. Hypomanic episodes have similar or milder symptoms and last at least four days. In *bipolar II disorder* there is a history of hypomanic as well as major depressive episodes. In *cyclothymia*, both milder hypomanic and depressive symptoms appear for most of the time over a period of at least two years.

Other mood disorders include depression related to medical illness, substance use or medication, or with an association to the menstrual cycle, or appearance during the winter months (seasonal affective disorder).

Here we will not dwell on specific diagnoses found in the people described in these chapters, as the purpose of this book is somewhat different: to tell the stories of these creative individuals, and to try and give a sense of what they were like and how their accomplishments came in the context of troubled lives. For this reason we have emphasized symptoms, what they experienced, rather than diagnoses which have been retrospectively attached to them. We will make a few general thoughts about psychiatric illnesses and creativity, with suggestions for further reading. The overall theme is that commenting on the presence of an illness alone may be of limited helpfulness in understanding an artist or writer's productivity; it may be better to consider the interaction of illness with personality traits and experiences. Additionally, as we will mention a little later, it seems important to take into account the influence of the historical context, for instance the moral codes, religious movements, and conflicts of the era.

Bipolar disorder:

If any single psychiatric condition seems to be found more frequently among writers and artists, it is likely some form of bipolar disorder. (Major depression, which is also often found, is discussed in the second part of this Addendum.) Some qualities of milder manic symptoms (hypomania) are related to better scores on creativity scales (Schuldberg, 1990). Jamison (1989) and others have noted the similarities of hypomania and the experience artists describe during periods of intense creativity—the energy, rapidity of thought, elation, and sense of grasping new connections. Close relatives of persons with bipolar illness generally score higher on measures of the ability to think creatively (Richards et al., 1988). In considering a possible relationship of bipolar disorder and creativity, two things come to mind:

1. Firstly, anyone who has witnessed a person in the midst of a full-blown manic episode will recognize that the degree of agitation, distractibility and disorganization of thinking makes it hard to generate the focus and structure needed to create great art. The artist Ellen Forney, put it this way: 'When I was manic, I didn't have enough focus. When I was depressed, I was so squashed.' (Forney, 2012, and quoted in Klein, 2017). For this reason, it has often been suggested that the type of mood disorder associated with creativity is bipolar II disorder, characterized by episodes of depression alternating after periods of normal functioning with shorter and less severe episodes of hypomania. These are more likely to be experienced as pleasurable, and can be associated with increased performance (APA, 2021).

    Some have argued that it is more useful to think of a spectrum of bipolar disorders, in a debate that harkens back to the nineteenth century roots of modern psychiatric diagnosis (Reddy, 2012). Regardless of whether one thinks of it as a group of several discrete diagnoses or a continuous gradient, the thing to keep in mind is that true manic episodes as seen in bipolar I disorder seem less likely to be associated with great art, and any relationship with creativity is more likely to be with a less severe form of bipolar mood disorder. Persons with bipolar II disorder are often found to have concurrent anxiety or substance use disorders, which can complicate the picture and which are often seen in writers and artists. Donald Goodwin (1988) has argued that a genetic tendency for bipolar illness may be the common link between creativity in writing and alcoholism.

2. If some form of bipolar disorder were to contribute to the making of great art, it of itself is likely not sufficient. About 2.8 percent of adults have had an episode of bipolar disorder in the past year, and 4.4 percent will experience it during their lifetime (NIMH, 2017). Clearly this is much more frequent than the number of persons who are outstanding artists. It seems more likely that something else is missing. If one route to creativity is aided by a form of bipolar disorder, it would probably involve an interaction with pre-existing cognitive skills and personality traits, for instance focus, commitment, the ability to apply structure to a work, and imagination. We will suggest other traits, as they come up, in later parts of this Addendum.

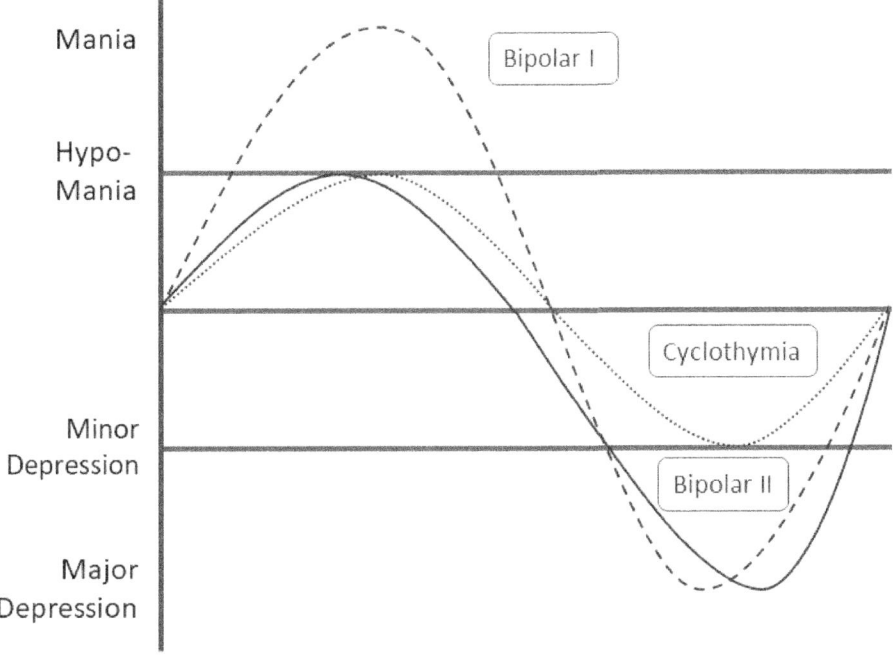

Figure A-1: *One of the ways to conceptualize the relationship of bipolar I, bipolar II, and cyclothymic disorders.*

Personality traits and disorders:

Studies of artists and writers have often found that they tend to score high on measures of a cluster of personality traits known as schizotypy (Burch et al., 2006; Nettle, 2006; Nelson and Rawlings, 2010). People with schizotypal qualities are thought to be isolated and distant, due to discomfort in social groups and difficulty with forming relationships. Additionally they may have perceptual distortions such as catching glimpses of something elusive at the edge of their vision, other illusions, or sensing that an absent person is there with them. These are often lumped together under the euphemism of 'unusual experiences'. Possible examples we have seen in this book might include the spacial transformations in Gogol's story 'A Terrible Vengeance', in which the geographically impossible takes place, and people in Kiev are suddenly able to see both the Crimea and the Carpathian Mountains. One could speculate whether Darwin's mind was naturally predisposed to accept Charles Lyell's notion of the earth being in constant flux, with coastlines shifting and seaside fossils appearing in the mountains over geological time. Persons with schizotypal personality disorder also often have unusual beliefs, including ideas, for instance, that they can read other's thoughts or have other special powers. They frequently have major mood disorders and histories of drug abuse and dependence (Bornstein et al., 1988).

The families of persons with schizotypal personality disorder tend to have a higher rate of schizophrenia, and there is some evidence of common genetic features between the two. Currently, the DSM-V (American Psychiatric Association, 2013), the standard reference of psychiatric diagnoses, has a category for 'schizotypal personality disorder', which is considered distinct from schizophrenia. In individuals with schizotypal personality disorder, the delusions and hallucinations are generally not as intense, and unlike persons with schizophrenia, they often can be persuaded that some of their distortions do not fit generally accepted reality.

There are also individuals who have many of the traits of schizotypal personality disorder but do not meet the full formal criteria. Just as it has often been thought that the very dramatic manic episodes of bipolar I disorder may be too disruptive for artistic creation, so that the less severe bipolar II might be more evident in artists, some researchers think that this milder form of schizotypal personality disorder is associated with creativity. It is often referred to as 'schizotypal personality' (Carson, 2011).

What are personality disorders?

Personality traits are habits in the way we think or relate, which persist relatively unchanged over long periods of time. When these traits become so conspicuous, rigid and enduring that they cause distress and impair functioning, they may be considered personality disorders. They often develop in early adulthood, though evidence of them may appear much earlier, and often persist throughout one's life. In general, genetic factors appear to play as much as a 50% role in their manifestation.

Schizotypal personality disorder includes some of the features which, in stronger form and in the context of loss of a sense of reality (psychosis) are seen in schizophrenia. It is one of 10 types of personality disorders recognized in the standardized compilation of psychiatric diagnoses, the DSM-V.

The notion that there is a relation of schizotypal qualities to creativity certainly carries an intuitive appeal. The novelist E.F. Doctorow, for instance, claimed that 'Writing is a socially acceptable form of schizophrenia' (Plimpton, 1986). It is not clear that he meant this literally, but it points to a widespread sense that writers are unusual people who may see things differently, and have unusual ways of thinking. The Andreasen study (1987) did not find an increase in schizophrenia in the relatives of writers, though for all of its many virtues it should be remembered that it involved only a small group of subjects. One study found that poets and artists have as high a rate of 'unusual experiences' as patients with schizophrenia, but differ in other ways, notably not sharing the inability to experience pleasure or decreased ability to act on their desires seen in the patients (Nettle, 2006). They were more likely to engage in 'divergent thinking', leading off into new, often original directions (Runco, 2011), compared to mathematicians, who displayed convergent thinking (using accepted rules and logic to solve problems). In a sense, this study follows in a tradition emphasized in the 1990s by Albert Rothenberg of Harvard University, who suggested that both creative persons and schizophrenics engage in 'translogical thinking', though there is a borderline between the beneficial aspects in the former, and what he described as the unproductive and 'impoverished' thinking of the latter (Rothenberg, 1990).

Another study found that a group of 100 artists and writers were more likely to display what is known as 'positive schizotypy', as well as other qualities including mood disturbances, neuroticism and openness to experience (Nelson and Rawlings, 2010). The features of schizotypy tended to be similar to what is seen in the creative process, such as 'distinct experience', 'absorption', 'anxiety' and

Dealing with too much information.

Each of us is constantly taking in large amounts of sensory information, which may make it difficult to focus on a particular subject or task. In order to make it possible to focus, a selective attention process sometimes referred to as 'latent inhibition' learns to weed out materials that seem irrelevant. It has been speculated that in schizotypy, this ability may be compromised, so that the mind is flooded with an excess of information. The result, for instance, might be the perceptual distortions or hallucinations in schizotypy (Carson, 2011). This has sometimes been viewed as a negative thing, perhaps being involved in the distractibility seen in schizophrenics. Others suggest that in milder form in schizotypy, it may facilitate creativity (Nelson and Rawlings, 2010). As we will see later in this section, it has also been speculated that depending on what other resources a person may have, it may predispose to either mental illness or creativity (Carson, 2011 and 2014).

'power/pleasure'. (A good example of immersion and intensity of experience may be reflected in Gogol's vivid description of the Dnieper River quoted in Chapter two.) The implication taken by Nelson and Rawlings was that the focus on current experience, absorption and pleasure in a project seen in positive schizotypy may lead to 'flow-type states' of creativity. This may be facilitated by a decrease in the normal filtering out of many sensory inputs and impressions as extraneous, so that conscious attention is exposed to a wider variety of materials, perhaps giving a fresh awareness and richness to current experience.

Although these data suggest that schizotypal personality disorder—or some of its features—might contribute to creative acts, it's important to remember that its frequency leads to the same limitation as bipolar disorder. A person has about a 3.9 percent likelihood of developing it during their lifetime (Pulay et al., 2009); clearly this many people do not all become great artists. It seems more likely that depending on what other qualities and resources a person has, it might predispose to a wide range of kinds of life, from a lonely, anxious, and less productive existence on the one hand, to a flow-fueled and expressive one on the other.

Signs of schizotypal personality disorder

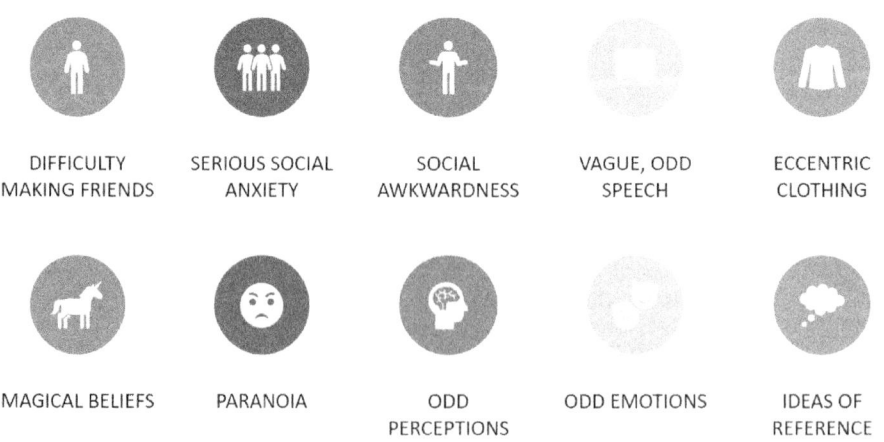

Figure A-2: *Schizotypal personality disorder.*

Psychological vulnerabilities and resources:

The notion that a decreased ability to filter out extraneous sensory information is associated with artistic expression suggests that in some situations a weakness or vulnerability may turn out to be an asset in individuals who have compensating strengths in processing information. The idea of the artist as a person who combines both vulnerabilities and strengths was explored from a somewhat different direction by Zorana Ivcevic, a psychologist at Yale University. She was struck by Frank Barron's description of creative individuals, quoted at the beginning of this chapter, particularly the thought that they are 'occasionally crazier yet adamantly saner' than most people. She hypothesized that creativity might be related to a particular combination of psychological vulnerabilities and resources. In her study one fourth of a research population of over 600 persons, equally divided into artists (faculty members at fine arts schools) and non-artists, had average psychological vulnerabilities such as depression, anxiety or susceptibility to stress, as well as an average amount of resources to deal with them such as hopefulness, ego resilience and a sense of well-being (Ivcevic et al., 2020a). Although greater vulnerability was often associated with having less resources, there was also a smaller group (9.4 percent) who had both high vulnerability as well as high resources. Interestingly, this pattern was more common in artists (16.2 percent) compared to non-artists (3.2 percent).

Ivcevic et al. speculated on the possibility that performing creative acts is a way by which artists deal with their vulnerabilities. In a sense this is a modern reformulation of an idea which in another context goes back to Sigmund Freud: that artists use creativity to deal with troubling thoughts, and in the process produce socially acceptable results instead of neurotic symptoms. Creativity, then, was seen as a kind of defense mechanism (Freud, 1908). Ultimately, though, the appeal of the more contemporary notion of high vulnerabilities matched with high resources suffers from the same caveat as with bipolar disorder and schizotypy—its high frequency. It has been found in about one-tenth of a research population (Ivcevic et al., 2020a; Ivcevic 2020b), and hence is likely much more common than the appearance of the kinds of writers and artists we have described here.

Looking at this more broadly, roughly one in five Americans displays some form of mental illness in a given year (Center for Behavioral Health Statistics, 2016), and about nine percent may have personality disorders (Lenzenweger, 2007). All these illnesses and traits are far more common than the number of remarkably creative artists, suggesting that they may predispose to creativity, but by themselves are not adequate. It may be more probable that they are contributory, but need to be combined with other qualities as well.

How, then, to explain the potential relationship of mental disorders to productivity in some artists? One possibility is that there may be a threefold role. Let's look at each of these in turn:

1. **Mental disorders as a spur to creativity:** The role of mental disorders in stimulating expression could come from the intense experiences they can produce, whether distressing (as in anxiety disorders) or potentially euphoric or grandiose (as in bipolar II disorder). Sometimes the desire to express these experiences seems very overt, such as in 'The Scream', the famous painting by Edvard Munch, who suffered from severe anxiety. Among the writers we have discussed, a good example would be Melville's comparison of his moods to a soaring eagle, or the grandiosity of feeling leading him to say that he would need 50 scribes to write down all his ideas.

2. **Providing a setting for creative work:** At the same time, mental disorders or personality traits may provide a setting which aids the creative process. Darwin recognized that the solitude of living in a remote village in Kent, avoiding professional meetings and visitors when possible, contributed to his work. Emily Dickinson's isolation, to the degree of speaking to visitors only from behind a closed door, may be considered a sign of illness, but also provided an environment for work with minimal disruption.

3. **Facilitating the creative process:** To summarize much of what we have presented above, some of the qualities of schizotypy such as absorption in new experiences and the ability to derive pleasure from them have been postulated to lead to 'flow-type' states; a tendency toward divergent thinking and having

'unusual experiences' have also been thought to be part of the creative process. In addition to openness to new experiences, being vulnerable in many ways—by experiencing anxiety, stress or depressed mood—may, when coupled with matching strengths, aid in creativity. Hypomanic states in bipolar II disorder may provide the energy, passionate feelings, and willingness to see new connections which contribute to making art. These remain speculations but are one way of putting together what we have seen from the lives of the writers presented here, as well as the results of studies of mental illness and creativity.

Are creativity and mental illness the results of a shared vulnerability?

It is also possible that mental illness or particular personality traits tend to occur together with artistic expression but that they do not necessarily drive each other; instead, it may be that they share a likelihood of appearing from a common, more basic source. This idea is known as the 'shared vulnerability model', in which Harvard psychologist Shelley H. Carson suggested that some aspects of the way the brain processes incoming information might predispose to either illness or artistic expression (Carson, 2011). Having to grapple with a flood of unfiltered sensory impressions might be distressing to some individuals, while for others—especially those equipped with high-functioning processing abilities such as significant intelligence and working memory, flexibility and a drive for self-expression—it might provide richer material for creative thoughts.

Other features which have been speculated to predispose to either mental illness or creativity include a sensitivity to novelty, and 'neural hyperconnectivity', the linking of areas in the brain not typically as well connected (Carson, 2011 and 2014). Many questions remain unanswered, for instance, whether decreased filtering of information is something that can vary at different times in creative individuals, or whether it is a more lasting trait, as it seems to be in persons at risk for illness. The broader theme to keep in mind, however, is that some more basic—and perhaps genetically influenced—cognitive mechanisms may underlie both the possibilities for creative work and the liability to illness.

What about the healthier artists?

It is also good to remember that not all artists have the possible predisposing qualities we have been looking at. While Ivcevic et al. (2020a) found that artists were more likely to have a combination of high psychological vulnerabilities and high resources (16.2 percent), that means that 83.8 percent did not. Similarly in the Andreasen (1987) study of writers in Iowa, 43 percent had bipolar illness, so 57 percent did not (though some had other mood disorders). Artists as a group have not always been found to have higher measures of bipolar symptoms (Nelson and Rawlings, 2006; Pavrita et al., 2007), and conversely, bipolar patients may not score higher on measures of creative ability (Ghadirian et al., 2000). Jamison (1989) found that 38 percent of a group of British writers and artists had been treated for a mood disorder, which reminds us to be aware of the other 62 percent who had not. Thus, although writers and artists often seem more likely to have certain personality traits or illnesses than others, it is wise to be cautious when generalizing about them as a group.

In Summary:

As we described in the last paragraphs, then, the frequent—but not inevitable—occurrence together of mental illness and artistic creativity does not necessarily indicate that one influences the other. Rather, the association may be that they both may derive from a common vulnerability. Even if one were to facilitate the other, it is important to remember the limitations on what can be gained by viewing great artists through the lens of psychiatric disorders. Certainly one thing lacking when focusing on symptoms of a possible mental disorder is an understanding of the influence of the social milieu and major events of the times: how Melville, for instance, tried to salvage his writing career by turning to poetry about the Civil War, or how Emily Dickinson delved into her own sense of loss when writing about the wartime casualties. Another limitation is apparent from the frequent occurrence of the psychiatric conditions we mentioned, compared with the rare appearance of brilliant writers and artists in a league with Melville, Poe or Rossetti. It seems more likely that these disorders and personality traits could either inhibit or promote artistic expression depending on whether they are accompanied by other qualities. We've mentioned some of the qualities which might contribute to great art along the way; others might include curiosity, commitment, fluency, discipline, and other still-elusive factors. The lives portrayed in the book offer a glimpse of what can happen in the rare cases when they all come together.

REFERENCES for ADDENDUM (PART 1)

American Psychiatric Association: Diagnostic and statistical manual of mental disorders (DSM-5), Fifth edition, 2013.
https://www.psychiatry.org/psychiatrists/practice/dsm

American Psychiatric Association: What is bipolar disorder? (Reviewed by M. Howland and A. El Sehamy, January, 2021).
https://www.psychiatry.org/patients-families/bipolar-disorders/what-are-bipolar-disorders

Andreasen N.C.: Creativity and mental illness: prevalence rates in writers and their first-degree relatives. Am. J. Psychiat. 144: 1288-1292, 1987.
https://pubmed.ncbi.nlm.nih.gov/3499088/

Andreasen, N.C.: The relationship between creativity and mood disorders. Dialogues Clin. Neurosci. 10: 251-255, 2008.
https://pubmed.ncbi.nlm.nih.gov/18689294/

Barron, F.: *Creativity and psychological health: origins of personal vitality and creative freedom.* Van Nostrand, Princeton, N.J., 1963.

Borenstein, R.F. et al.: Schizotypal personality disorder in an outpatient population: incidence and clinical characteristics.
https://pubmed.ncbi.nlm.nih.gov/3384958/

Burch St. J. et al.: Schizotypy and creativity in visual artists. British Journal of Psychology 97: 139-280, 2006.
https://bpspsychub.onlinelibrary.wiley.com/doi/abs/10.1348/0007
12605X60030

Carson, S.H.: Creativity and psychopathology: a shared vulnerability model. Can. J. Psychiat. 56: 144-153, 2011.
https://pubmed.ncbi.nlm.nih.gov/21443821/

Carson, S: Leveraging the "mad genius" debate: why we need a neuroscience of creativity and psychopathology. Frontiers in Human Neuroscience.8: 771, 1014.
https://www.ncbi.nlm.nih.gov/pmc/articles/PMC4179620/

Center for Behavioral Health Statistics and Quality, Substance Abuse and Mental Health Services Administration: Key substance use and mental health indicators in the United States: Results from the 2015 National Survey on Drug Use and Health. Rockville, MD. 2016. Cited by Centers for Disease Control and Prevention,
https://www.cdc.gov/mentalhealth/learn/index.htm

Deshpande, N.S. et al.: The perpetual fragility of creeping hillslopes. Nature Communications 12: article number 3909 (2021).

https://www.nature.com/articles/s41467-021-23979-z

Forney, E.: *Marbles: mania, depression, Michelangelo, and me: a graphic memoir.* Avery, illustrated edition, 2012.
https://www.amazon.com/Marbles-Depression-Michelangelo-Graphic-Memoir/dp/1592407323?tag=thehuffingtop-20

Freud, S.: *Creative writers and daydreaming.* (1908).
https://static1.squarespace.com/static/5441df7ee4b02f59465d2869/t/588e9620e6f2e152d3ebcffc/1485739554918/Freud+-+Creative+Writers+and+Day+Dreaming%281%29.pdf

Ghadirian, A.-M., Gregoire, P., & Kosmidis, H. Creativity and the evolution of psychopathologies. Creativity Research Journal, 13(2), 145–148, 2000-2001.

Goodwin, D.W.: *Alcohol and the writer.* Andrews and McMeel, Kansas City and New York, 1988.

Ivcevic, Z., Grossman, E., & Ranjan, A. (2020a). Patterns of psychological vulnerabilities and resources in artists and nonartists. Psychology of Aesthetics, Creativity, and the Arts. Advance online publication.
https://doi.org/10.1037/aca0000309 Accessed March 2, 2021.

Ivcevic, Z.: The paradox of creativity: high psychological vulnerabilities and resources. Psychology of Aesthetics Creativity

and the Arts, April 2020, American Psychological Association (APA) 2020b.
https://www.growkudos.com/publications/10.1037%25252Faca0000309/reader

Jamison, K.R.: Mood disorders and patterns of creativity in British writers and artists. Psychiatry 52: 125, 1989.
https://doi.org/10.1080/00332747.1989.11024436

Klein, S.: What neuroscience has to say about the 'tortured genius'. Huffpost.com, updated 12/6/2017.
https://www.huffpost.com/entry/creativity-mental-illness-health_n_5695887 Accessed 7/8/21.

Langsdorf, W.B.: *Tranquility of mind.* New York, Putnam's Sons, 1900.

Lenzenweger MF, Lane MC, Loranger AW, Kessler RC. DSM-IV personality disorders in the National Comorbidity Survey Replication. *Biol Psychiatry.* 2007 Sep 15;62(6):553-64.
https://pubmed.ncbi.nlm.nih.gov/17217923/

Mendelson, W.B.: *Trial by fire: World War II and the founders of modern neuroscience and neuropsychopharmacology.* Pythagoras Press, 2020.
https://www.amazon.com/dp/B08X1MRVXJ

Nettle, D.: Schizotypy and mental health among poets, visual artists, and mathematicians. J. Res. Personality 40: 876-890, 2006.
https://www.sciencedirect.com/science/article/abs/pii/S00926566
05000620

Nelson, B. and Rawlings, D.: Relating schizotypy and personality to the phenomenology of creativity. Schizophrenia Bulletin 36: 388-399, 2010.
https://academic.oup.com/schizophreniabulletin/article/36/2/388
/1896891

NIMH: Bipolar disorder. Updated November, 2017; Accessed May 21, 2021..
https://www.nimh.nih.gov/health/statistics/bipolar-disorder

Pavrita, K.S. et al.: Creativity and mental health: a profile of writers and musicians. Indian. J. Psychiat. 49: 34-43, 2007.
https://www.ncbi.nlm.nih.gov/pmc/articles/PMC2899997/
Accessed 2/28/21.

Plimpton, G.: E.L. Doctorow, The art of fiction no. 94. The Paris Review 101, winter 1986.
https://www.theparisreview.org/interviews/2718/the-art-of-fiction-no-94-e-l-doctorow

Pulay, A.J. et al.: Prevalence, correlates, disability, and comorbidity of DSM-IV schizotypal personality disorder: results from the wave 2 national epidemiologic survey on alcohol and related conditions. Prim. Care Companion J. Clin. Psychiatry 11: 53-67, 2009.

https://www.ncbi.nlm.nih.gov/pmc/articles/PMC2707116/

Reddy, M.S.: The bipolar spectrum. Ind. J. Psychological Med. 34: 1-4, 2012.

https://www.ncbi.nlm.nih.gov/pmc/articles/PMC3361834/

Richards, R. et al.: Creativity in manic depressives, cyclothymes, their normal relatives, and control subjects. J. Abnormal Psychology. 97: 281-288, 1988.

Rothenberg, A.: *Creativity and madness: new findings and old stereotypes.* Johns Hopkins University Press, Baltimore, 1990.

Runco, M.A.: Divergent thinking. Encyclopedia of creativity (Second Edition, 2011).

https://www.sciencedirect.com/topics/psychology/divergent-thinking

Schuldberg, D.: Schizotypal and hypomanic traits, creativity, and psychological health. Creativity Research Journal. 3: 218-230, 1990.

Taiylor, C.L.: Creativity and mood disorder: a systematic review and meta-analysis. Perspectives on psychological science. 12: 1040-1076, 2017.

https://doi.org/10.1177/1745691617699653

UpToDate: Diagnostic criteria for minor depression. UpToDate Inc., 2021.

https://www.uptodate.com/contents/image?imageKey=PSYCH/10 6958

Part 2

Abraham Lincoln: depression, creativity and leadership

Abraham Lincoln's tendency toward what was then called 'melancholy' was well known by his neighbors in New Salem, Illinois. In his mid-twenties, after a woman to whom he felt close died of typhoid fever, he led an isolated life, spent long periods of time alone in the woods with his gun, and wrote gloomy poetry. At one point, the local justice of the peace and his wife convinced him to move in with them, but after a couple of weeks of being cared for, he remained morose. Though he occasionally sought merriment with his friends, he confided to one colleague that his mood was such that he dared not carry a knife.

Five years later in 1840, the young politician was so troubled that neighbors removed all the razors and sharp objects from his home. He requested help from a doctor, with whom he began to spend several hours a day. At one point, records from a Springfield pharmacy indicated that he sought pharmacologic relief with various medicines including sedatives, camphor and mercury-based 'blue mass' pills. (The latter, which he later discontinued, contained roughly 100 times the modern EPA guidelines for mercury; it has been speculated that mercury poisoning may also have contributed to his depressive symptoms, and anger outbursts, as well as tremor and difficulty walking.) Feelings of failure and doom, as well as fatigue interspersed with agitation, and thoughts of death haunted him his whole life, even as he struggled with the great issues of his day, presided over the foremost crisis in the country's history, and ultimately saved his nation (Shenk, 2005).

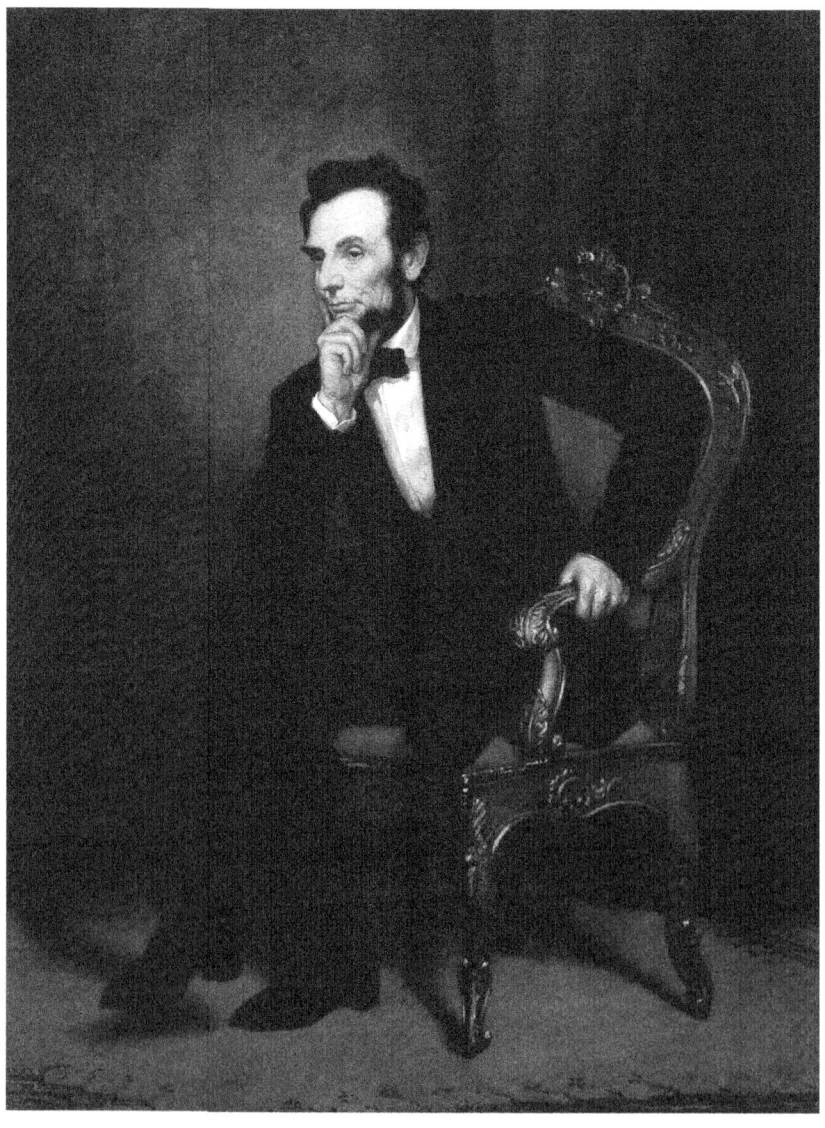

Figure A-3: Abraham Lincoln, *by George Peter Alexander Healy, 1869. Healy (1813-1894) was one of the most well-known American artists at the time. He was working in Paris when he painted this picture following an 1869 act of Congress authorizing a portrait of Lincoln. It now is displayed in the State Dining Room of the White House.*

The list of historical political and military figures who appear to have suffered from depression goes on and on, including Lincoln's contemporaries Benjamin Disraeli and William T. Sherman, later notables such as Winston Churchill, writers more recent than those in this book (Ernest Hemingway, J.K. Rowling) and modern celebrities (Jim Carrey, Eminem, Anne Hathaway). Articles about the possible relation of depression to success in politics or the arts have taken two general views—that these people were able to overcome their depression and go on to greatness, or alternatively that something about their mood disorder aided them in the process. One article on Lincoln, for instance, described three stages which he went through—fear, engagement, and transcendence—and argued that 'Whatever greatness Lincoln achieved cannot be explained as a triumph over personal suffering. Rather, it must be accounted an outgrowth of the same system that produced that suffering... Lincoln didn't do great work because he solved the problem of his melancholy; the problem of his melancholy was all the more fuel for the fire of his great work' (Shenk, 2005). We will look at this latter possibility, considering two types of arguments, that: 1. The ubiquity and evolutionary persistence of depression suggest that it might be useful; and 2. There are possible cognitive mechanisms by which depression might have positive value.

The evolutionary argument for depression:

In the first part of the Addendum we touched on the frequency of mood disorders (primarily bipolar disorder) while making the point that they occur much more often than the number of great artists. Here we'll look at a different issue, focusing on depression—whether its persistent high frequency across evolutionary time indicates that it may be beneficial in some way. Even though many of the features of depression such as fatigue and decreased appetite and libido would seem to have negative evolutionary value, some have argued that its ubiquity—it is experienced by about seven percent of Americans in any given year—suggests some selective advantage. It's important to remember, though, that evolution has allowed the continuance of other states which seem less likely to be helpful for survival, such as psychopathy. On the one hand, it is possible that psychopathy persists because it is relatively rare, with a prevalence of less than one percent ('frequency-dependent selection'), but this is hardly the case for depression. On the other hand, one explanation which has been applied to psychopathy is that it could result from such a large number of mutations that any single one is less likely to be under evolutionary pressure; this could be applied to depression, in which genomic studies have found that as many as 102 independent variants and 269 genes (Howard et al., 2019) may play a role. It is difficult, then, for natural selection to eliminate a trait with such complex origins.

Even if depression is associated with greater adaptivity, it may be that it is not depression *per se*, but some other unknown trait to which it is genetically linked, that has positive value. Or it could be that depression had some value in a past age or some specific situation that is now less applicable, and in that sense is similar to sickle cell disease in modern Western society. All in all, it should not be a foregone conclusion that the ubiquity of depression means that it has been favored by evolution.

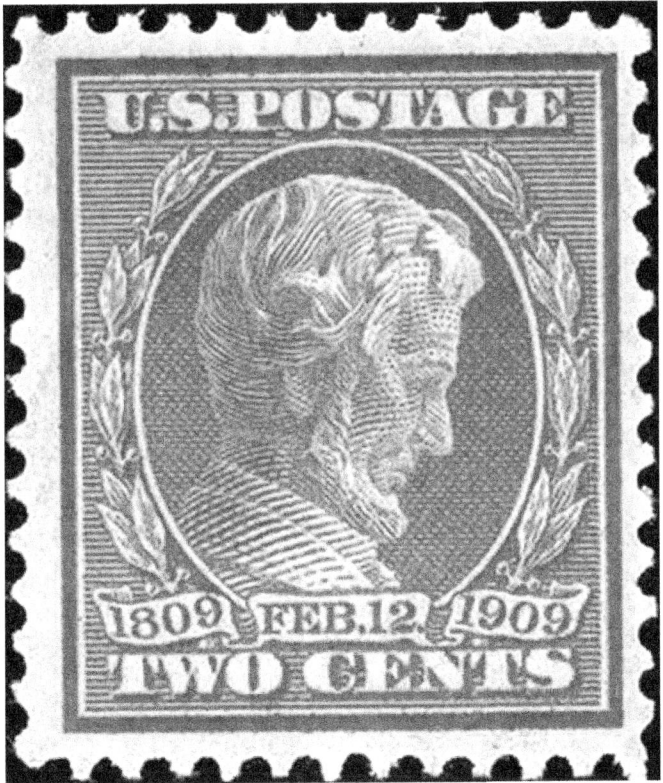

Figure A-4: *Postage stamp depicting Abraham Lincoln, 1909*

Potentially helpful cognitive traits in depression:

At least two kinds of cognitive traits have been taken to support some positive aspects of depression. They suggest that either the ruminations typical of depression, or a potentially more realistic assessment of situations, may have value in problem-solving. Let's look at each of these:

Ruminations: The notion that dwelling on repetitive thoughts may be useful has gained support from an fMRI study showing changes in brain networks associated with this activity (Zhang et al., 2020). The "analytical rumination hypothesis" suggests that ruminations can lead to useful reasoning, first in a causal analysis and then in a problem-solving analysis. The implication is that ruminations can help a person come up with explanations and solutions for an unhappy event. There are some data that problem-solving analysis is associated with decreased persistence of depressive symptoms (Sevcikova et al., 2020).

Counter-arguments would be that this view works best when depression seems tied to a particular trauma, and may more likely be a healthy response in a person who is sad after a specific upset; it is less clear how it might work in seemingly paralyzing severe depression, chronic depression, post-stroke depression, or mood disorders of old age (Lehrer, 2010). One review reported that among those who study evolutionary psychology, there is a pretty much even split over whether rumination is adaptive; it suggests that supporters are more likely to be non-clinicians, while clinicians, who have witnessed patients who seem stuck in ongoing non-constructive circular thinking, are more skeptical (Kennair et al., 2017).

Another way of viewing it is that we need to bear in mind the distinction between sadness, a universal human experience in response to painful events, and major depression, in which a despondent mood dominates one's life for at least two weeks, and is associated with decreased functioning, cognitive changes, and a host of physical symptoms. It might be that ruminations are more likely to be useful when one is sad, but that in major depression they are more likely to be circular and non-constructive. In major depression, then, ruminations might be part of a constellation of cognitive changes which are generally unhelpful, including alterations in memory, attention and decision-making.

More realistic assessment of situations: A second argument as to how depression might be adaptive suggests that persons with depression benefit from what is known as "depressive realism." In one often-cited study, depressed and non-depressed students were given problems on a computer and asked to what degree they felt their actions were related to a light flashing on the screen. Non-depressed subjects tended to overestimate their responsibility when light flashing was frequent and considered desirable, and to underestimate it when lights were considered undesirable. In contrast, depressed persons had much more realistic assessments of the degree to which their actions were responsible for the lights flashing (Alloy and Abramson, 1979).

The degree to which depressive realism could play a role is not firmly established. One large analysis of available studies concluded that overall there was "a small depressive realism effect." On the other hand, the authors noted that the findings were more likely to be positive in studies that lacked objective measures of realism and relied more on self-report (Moore and Fresco, 2012).

In summary:

Depression's ubiquity does not necessarily argue that evolution has favored it as an advantageous trait. Though it is an attractive idea that goes back to antiquity, modern studies have had mixed results on whether there is a relationship between major depression and creativity. The hypothesis that ruminations in depression lead to problem-solving is controversial, and may be of limited applicability. A second notion is depressive realism, but its effect is small and whether it is seen at all is highly dependent on the methodology of the studies.

It's important, then, to distinguish between sadness or depressed feelings in response to specific difficult experiences on the one hand, and major depressive disorder on the other. It seems possible that we have a built-in response to specific stressful situations which sometimes can be of help in assessing problems and leading to solutions. It also seems possible that some people such as Lincoln found ways to harness their distress and use it to spur a drive for achievement. But this is different from arguing that major depression is an often-helpful state, or that any potential upside compensates for the suffering it involves.

REFERENCES for ADDENDUM (PART 2)

Alloy, L.B. and Abramson, L.Y.: Judgment of contingency in depressed and nondepressed students: sadder but wiser? J. Experimental Psychol. General 108: 441-485, 1979.
https://pubmed.ncbi.nlm.nih.gov/528910/

Howard, D.M. et al.: Genome—wide meta-analysis of depression identifies 102 independent variants and highlights the importance of the prefrontal brain regions. Nat. Neurosci. 22: 343-352, 2019.
https://pubmed.ncbi.nlm.nih.gov/30718901/

Kennair L.E.O., Kleppestø T.H., Larsen S.M., Jørgensen B.E.G. (2017) Depression: Is Rumination Really Adaptive?. In: Shackelford T., Zeigler-Hill V. (eds) The Evolution of Psychopathology. Evolutionary Psychology. Springer, Cham.
https://doi.org/10.1007/978-3-319-60576-0_3

Lehrer, J.: Comments by Peter Kramer in 'Depression's Upside', New York Times, February 25, 2010.

Moore, M.T. and Fresco, D.M.: Depressive realism: a meta-analytic review. Clin. Psychol. Rev. 32: 496-509, 2012.

https://doi.org/10.1016/j.cpr.2012.05.004

Sevcikova, M. et al.: Testing the analytical rumination hypothesis: exploring the longitudinal effects of problem solving analysis on depression. Front. Psychol. 02 July, 2020.
https://doi.org/10.3389/fpsyg.2020.01344

Shenk, J.W.: Lincoln's great depression. The Atlantic, October 2005. https://www.theatlantic.com/magazine/archive/2005/10/lincolns-great-depression/304247/ Accessed 2/28/21.

Zhang, R. et al.: Rumination network dysfunction in major depression: a brain connectome study. Prog. Neuro-Psychopharmacol and Biol. Psychiat. 98, March 2020.
https://doi.org/10.1016/j.pnpbp.2019.109819

Portions of Part 2 of the Addendum are adapted from the author's blog in *Psychology Today* on March 1 and April 1, 2021. Portions of the chapter on Herman Melville are adapted from the author's blog in *Psychology Today* on August 6, 2021.

PICTURE CREDITS

Cover Illustration: (The Raven) U.S. Lithograph Co, Cincinnati and Russell-Morgan Print, New York, in Wikimedia Commons, which states 'This media file is in the public domain in the United States. This applies to U.S. works where the copyright has expired, often because its first publication occurred prior to January 1, 1926, and if not then due to lack of notice or renewal.'

Fig. 1-1: (Typee) Augustus Burnham Shute, in Typee, 1892, in Wikimedia Commons, which states 'This media file is in the public domain in the United States. This applies to U.S. works where the copyright has expired, often because its first publication occurred prior to January 1, 1926, and if not then due to lack of notice or renewal.'

Figure 2-1: (drawing of Nikolai Gogol) Emmanuil Dmitriev-Mamonov, 1850-1860s, in Wikimedia Commons, which states 'This work is in the public domain in the United States because it was published (or registered with the U.S. Copyright Office) before January 1, 1926.'

Figure 2-2: (stamp of 'The Government Inspector') Scanned and processed by Andrew Krizhanovsky, in Wikimedia Commons, which states 'This work is not an object of copyright according to article 1259 of Book IV of the Civil Code of the Russian Federation No. 230-FZ of December 18, 2006.'

Figure 2-3: (stamp of 'The Overcoat') Scanned and processed by Andrew Krizhanovsky, in Wikimedia Commons, which states 'This work is not an object of copyright according to article 1259 of Book IV of the Civil Code of the Russian Federation No. 230-FZ of December 18, 2006.'

Figure 2-4: (Gogol Bordello) Brian Hayden Safdie, in Wikimedia Commons, which states 'This file is licensed under the Creative Commons Share-Alike 2.0 generic license.'

Figure 3-1: (The Sleeper) W. Heath Robinson, 1900, in Wikimedia Commons, which states 'This work is in the public domain in its country of origin and other countries and areas where the copyright term is the author's life plus 70 years or fewer.' In the United States: 'This file has been identified as being free of known restrictions under copyright law, including all related and neighboring rights.'

Figure 3-2: (Contes Grotesques by Edgar Allan Poe) Muschio Di Quercia, in Wikimedia Commons, which states 'This file is licensed under the Creative Commons Share-Alike 4.0 international license.'

Figure 4-1: (Proserpine) Dante Gabriel Rossetti, in Wikimedia Commons, which states 'This work is in the public domain in its country of origin and other countries and areas where the copyright term is the author's life plus 100 years or fewer.' In the United States: 'This file has been identified as being free of known restrictions under copyright law, including all related and neighboring rights.'

Figure 4-2: (Dante's Dream) Art UK, in Wikimedia Commons, which states 'The author died in 1882, so this work is in the public domain of its country of origin and other countries and areas where the copyright term is the author's life plus 100 years or fewer.' 'This work is in the public domain in the United States because it was published (or registered with the U.S. Copyright Office) before January 1, 1926.'

Figure 5-1: (The Homestead) Daderot, from Wikimedia Commons, which states 'I, the copyright holder of this work, release this work into the public domain. This applies worldwide.'

Figure 5-2: (Homestead) Tomwsulcer, from Wikimedia Commons, which states 'This file is made available under the Creative Commons CC0 1.0 Universal Public domain dedication.'

Figure 6-1: (HMS Beagle) C. Martens and T. Landseer, in Wikimedia Commons, which states 'This file is made available under the Creative Commons CC0 1.0 Universal Public domain dedication.'

Figure 6-2: (Map of the voyage of the Beagle) Kipala, Samsara, and Dave Souza (Semhur) in Wikimedia Commons, which states 'This file is licensed under the Creative Commons Attribution-Share Alike 4.0 International, 3.0 unported, 2.5 generic, 2.0 generic, and 1.0 generic license.'

Figure 6-3: (Darwin's study) In *Charles Darwin, His Life and Work* by Charles Frederick Holder, 1891. From The Wellcome Collection. License: Public Domain Mark.

Figure 6-4: (Darwin's sketch of evolutionary tree) In Darwin, C., 'The First Notebook on Transmutation of Species', 1837, on display at the Museum of Natural History, Manhattan. From Wikipedia Commons, which states 'This work is in the public domain in its country of origin and other countries and areas where the copyright term is the author's life plus 70 years or fewer.' 'This work is in the public domain in the United States because it was published (or registered with the U.S. Copyright Office) before January 1, 1926.' Reference for the interpretation of handwriting, taken from the same page in Wikipedia Commons, is found in the figure caption in the text.

Figure A-1: (graph of bipolar disorders) Adapted from Blacktc, from Wikimedia Commons, which states 'This file is licensed under the Creative Commons Attribution 4.0 International license.'

Figure A-2: (schizotypal personality disorder) MissLunaRose 12, from Wikipedia Commons, which states 'This file is licensed under the Creative Commons Attribution-Share Alike 4.0 International license.'

Figure A-3: (Abraham Lincoln) George Peter Alexander Healy's *Abraham Lincoln*, from Wikipedia Commons, which states 'This work is in the public domain of its country of origin and other countries and areas where the copyright term is the author's life plus 100 years or fewer.' 'This work is in the public domain in the United States because it was published (or registered with the U.S. Copyright Office) before January 1, 1926.'

Figure A-4: (Lincoln stamp) U.S. Post Office Gwillhickers, in Wikimedia Commons, which states 'This work is in the public domain in the United States because it is a work prepared by an officer or employee of the United States Government as part of that person's official duties under there terms of Title 17, Chapter 1, Section 105 of the US code.'

Printed in Great Britain
by Amazon